HISTORY OF BRITISH INTENSIVE CARE, c.1950–c.2000

The transcript of a Witness Seminar held by the Wellcome Trust Centre for the History of Medicine at UCL, The Wellcome Trust, on 16 June 2010

Edited by L A Reynolds and E M Tansey

Volume 42   2011

D1439467

©The Trustee of the Wellcome Trust, London, 2011

First published by Queen Mary, University of London, 2011

The History of Modern Biomedicine Research Group is funded by the Wellcome Trust, which is a registered charity, no. 210183.

ISBN 978 090223 875 6

All volumes are freely available online at www.history.qmul.ac.uk/research/modbiomed/
wellcome_witnesses/

Please cite as: Reynolds L A, Tansey E M. (eds) (2011) *History of British intensive care, c.1950–c.2000*. Wellcome Witnesses to Twentieth Century Medicine, vol. 42. London: Queen Mary, University of London.

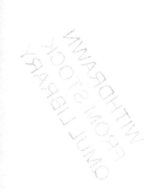

CONTENTS

ILLUSTRATIONS AND CREDITS

ABBREVIATIONS

AC	alternating current
ARDS	acute respiratory distress syndrome
APACHE	Acute Physiology, Age, Chronic Health Evaluation critical illness scoring system
BACCN	British Association of Critical Care Nurses
BBC	British Broadcasting Corporation
BTA	Been to America
CoBaTrICE	Competency Based Training programme in Intensive Care Medicine for Europe
CVP	central venous pressure
DC	direct current
DIPEx	Database of Individual Personal Experiences
ECCO$_2$R	extra-corporeal carbon dioxide removal
ECG	electrocardiogram
ECMO	extracorporeal membrane oxygenation
ENB	English National Board for Nursing, Midwifery and Health Visiting
ENT	ear, nose and throat
FICM	Faculty of Intensive Care Medicine
GGHB	Greater Glasgow Health Board
GMC	General Medical Council
HBN27	Hospital Building Note 27 (Health Building Note after 1992)
HDU	high dependency unit
HP	house physician
ICNARC	Intensive Care National Audit and Research Centre
ICS	Intensive Care Society

ICU/ITU	intensive care/therapy unit
IPPR	intermittent positive pressure respiration
IPPV	intermittent positive pressure ventilation
ITU	intensive therapy unit
JBCNS	Joint Board of Clinical Nursing Studies
MGH	Massachusetts General Hospital, Boston, Massachusetts
NICG	Nursing Intensive Care Group
NIPPV	non-invasive positive pressure ventilation
NMC	Nursing and Midwifery Council
PAC	pulmonary artery catheter
PCO_2	arterial blood partial pressure of carbon dioxide
PO_2	arterial blood partial pressure of oxygen
PRCP	President of the Royal College of Physicians of London
RAF	Royal Air Force
RAP	resident assistant physician
RCN	Royal College of Nursing
RCP	Royal College of Physicians of London
SCCM	Society of Critical Care Medicine
TEG	thrombo-elastograph monitoring equipment
UKCC	UK Central Council for Nursing, Midwifery and Health Visiting

WITNESS SEMINARS:
MEETINGS AND PUBLICATIONS [1]

In 1990 the Wellcome Trust created a History of Twentieth Century Medicine Group, associated with the Academic Unit of the Wellcome Institute for the History of Medicine, to bring together clinicians, scientists, historians and others interested in contemporary medical history. Among a number of other initiatives the format of Witness Seminars, used by the Institute of Contemporary British History to address issues of recent political history, was adopted, to promote interaction between these different groups, to emphasize the potential benefits of working jointly, and to encourage the creation and deposit of archival sources for present and future use. In June 1999 the Governors of the Wellcome Trust decided that it would be appropriate for the Academic Unit to enjoy a more formal academic affiliation and turned the Unit into the Wellcome Trust Centre for the History of Medicine at UCL from 1 October 2000 to 30 September 2010. The History of Twentieth Century Medicine Group has been part of the School of History, Queen Mary, University of London, since October 2010, as the History of Modern Biomedicine Research Group, which the Wellcome Trust continues to fund.

The Witness Seminar is a particularly specialized form of oral history, where several people associated with a particular set of circumstances or events are invited to come together to discuss, debate, and agree or disagree about their memories. To date, the History of Twentieth Century Medicine Group has held nearly 50 such meetings, most of which have been published, as listed on pages pages xv–xix.

Subjects are usually proposed by, or through, members of the Programme Committee of the Group, which includes professional historians of medicine, practising scientists and clinicians, and once an appropriate topic has been agreed, suitable participants are identified and invited. This inevitably leads to further contacts, and more suggestions of people to invite. As the organization of the meeting progresses, a flexible outline plan for the meeting is devised, usually with assistance from the meeting's chairman, and some participants are invited to 'set the ball rolling' on particular themes, by speaking for a short period to initiate and stimulate further discussion.

---

[1] The following text also appears in the 'Introduction' to recent volumes of *Wellcome Witnesses to Twentieth Century Medicine* as listed on pages xv–xix.

Each meeting is fully recorded, the tapes are transcribed and the unedited transcript is immediately sent to every participant. Each is asked to check his or her own contributions and to provide brief biographical details. The editors turn the transcript into readable text, and participants' minor corrections and comments are incorporated into that text, while biographical and bibliographical details are added as footnotes, as are more substantial comments and additional material provided by participants. The final scripts are then sent to every contributor, accompanied by forms assigning copyright to the Wellcome Trust. Copies of all additional correspondence received during the editorial process are deposited with the records of each meeting in archives and manuscripts, Wellcome Library, London.

As with all our meetings, we hope that even if the precise details of some of the technical sections are not clear to the non-specialist, the sense and significance of the events will be understandable. Our aim is for the volumes that emerge from these meetings to inform those with a general interest in the history of modern medicine and medical science; to provide historians with new insights, fresh material for study, and further themes for research; and to emphasize to the participants that events of the recent past, of their own working lives, are of proper and necessary concern to historians.

ACKNOWLEDGEMENTS

'British intensive care' was suggested as a suitable topic for a Witness Seminar by Dr Tony Gilbertson, Professor Iain Ledingham and Dr David Wright, who assisted us in planning the meeting. We are very grateful to them for that input and to Professor Peter Hutton for his excellent chairing of the occasion. We are particularly grateful to Professor Sir Ian Gilmore for writing the Introduction to the published proceedings. We thank Professors Ronald Bradley, Iain Ledingham and Sir Keith Sykes and Drs Margaret Branthwaite, Geoffrey Spencer and Joseph Stoddart for their help with the photographs; and to Ms Alice Nicholls, who is completing her PhD on the subject, for acting as reader and providing additional information. We are most grateful to Professor Sir Keith Sykes for his expert reading of the transcript. For permission to reproduce images included here, we thank the British Polio Fellowship, the Chartered Society of Physiotherapy and the Intensive Care Society. Permission was requested from the anaesthesia and critical care department, University of Newcastle upon Tyne, the East Liverpool Hospital Management Committee, Liverpool Regional Hospital Board and the Nuffield department of anaesthetics, University of Oxford, as copyright holders, but no reply was received. Additionally, we would like to thank Dr David Morrison, whom one of us (TT) met while travelling in Northern Russia on the way to Archangel. A dinner conversation in Yaroslavl revealed our respective professions and he generously agreed to comment on, and add to, the records of this meeting.

As with all our meetings, we depend a great deal on our colleagues at the Wellcome Trust to ensure their smooth running: the Audiovisual Department, Catering, Reception, Security and Wellcome Images; Mr Akio Morishima has supervised the design and production of this volume; we thank our indexer, Ms Liza Furnival, and our readers, Ms Fiona Plowman and Mrs Sarah Beanland. Mrs Debra Gee is our transcriber, and Mrs Wendy Kutner and Ms Stefania Crowther assisted us in running this meeting. Finally, we thank the Wellcome Trust for supporting this programme.

Tilli Tansey

Lois Reynolds

School of History, Queen Mary, University of London

VOLUMES IN THIS SERIES

All volumes are freely available online at www.history.qmul.ac.uk/research/ modbiomed/wellcome_witnesses

Hard copies of volumes 21–42 can be ordered from www.amazon.co.uk; www.amazon.com; and all good booksellers for £6/$10 each plus postage, using the ISBN.

UNPUBLISHED WITNESS SEMINARS

1994   **The early history of renal transplantation**

1994   **Pneumoconiosis of coal workers**
(partially published in volume 13, *Population-based research in south Wales*)

1995   **Oral contraceptives**

2003   **Beyond the asylum: Anti-psychiatry and care in the community**

2003   **Thrombolysis**
(partially published in volume 27, *Cholesterol, atherosclerosis and coronary disease in the UK, 1950–2000*)

2007   **DNA fingerprinting**

The transcripts and records of all Witness Seminars are held in archives and manuscripts, Wellcome Library, London, at GC/253.

OTHER PUBLICATIONS

Technology transfer in Britain: The case of monoclonal antibodies
Tansey E M, Catterall P P. (1993) *Contemporary Record* **9**: 409–44.

Monoclonal antibodies: A witness seminar on contemporary medical history
Tansey E M, Catterall P P. (1994) *Medical History* **38**: 322–7.

Chronic pulmonary disease in South Wales coalmines: An eye-witness account of the MRC surveys (1937–42)
P D'Arcy Hart, edited and annotated by E M Tansey. (1998)
Social History of Medicine **11**: 459–68.

Ashes to Ashes – The history of smoking and health
Lock S P, Reynolds L A, Tansey E M. (eds) (1998) Amsterdam: Rodopi BV,
228pp. ISBN 90420 0396 0 (Hfl 125) (hardback). Reprinted 2003.

Witnessing medical history. An interview with Dr Rosemary Biggs
Professor Christine Lee and Dr Charles Rizza (interviewers). (1998)
Haemophilia **4**: 769–77.

Witnessing the Witnesses: Pitfalls and potentials of the Witness Seminar in twentieth century medicine
Tansey E M, in Doel R, Søderqvist T. (eds) (2006) *Writing Recent Science: The historiography of contemporary science, technology and medicine.* London: Routledge: 260–78.

The Witness Seminar technique in modern medical history
Tansey E M, in Cook H J, Bhattacharya S, Hardy A. (eds) (2008) *History of the Social Determinants of Health: Global Histories, Contemporary Debates.* London: Orient Longman: 279–95.

Today's medicine, tomorrow's medical history
Tansey E M, in Natvig J B, Swärd E T, Hem E. (eds) (2009) *Historier om helse* (*Histories about Health,* in Norwegian). Oslo: *Journal of the Norwegian Medical Association:* 166–73.

INTRODUCTION

You might ask what a gastroenterologist is doing writing this foreword when his whole lifetime experience of intensive care medicine amounted to four months at St Thomas' Hospital in 1973, but it was a period that changed my life – for several reasons.

The 'Mead Job' was the most highly sought-after post for aspiring physicians (aspiring anaesthetists may have sought the post too, but very rarely passed Ron Bradley's critical assessment). The list of past SHO's on Mead since it opened about 1967 is a roll-call of honour in British medicine at St Thomas' – I know, because Ron sent me the list when I became PRCP).[1] I realised that I had little chance of getting the job – having failed to get a house physician post at St Thomas' (and my professorial surgical unit house officer post counted for nought) – and so I went to the Whittington Hospital, famous for its ability to get just about anyone through MRCP. This put me in the happy position, just ten months after finishing my house jobs, of applying to Mead with 'the membership' and this was sufficiently unusual for me to be allowed to fill an unexpected vacancy. After the most frightening fortnight of my life, thrown into the deep end, chance would have it that I was sent out of the front-line trenches to fill a two-month slot at the South-Western Hospital (London, SW9) where Geoffrey Spencer ran his internationally acclaimed unit for chronic respiratory failure – usually as a consequence of polio. Although we were 'on' 168 hours a week, the pace was slower and the clientele fascinating. Back to Mead ward two months later and I was able to complete unfinished business by asking out attractive staff nurse Douglas (now Lady Gilmore, see Figure 11) and apply successfully for a registrar post (successful only because Ron Bradley was on the committee and sitting next to David McBrien from Worthing Hospital, where the rotation started, no doubt telling him whom he should appoint). So my time as Mead SHO was cut short.

I would not have survived the 12 months at Worthing without the Mead training – the sole medical registrar ran the intensive care unit (ICU) and the consultant anaesthetist in charge called in once a month whether it was needed or not! During the 12 months, Ron rang offering me a research post investigating the

---

[1] The list of SHOs serving on Mead ward, 1966 to 1994, from Professor Ronald Bradley will be deposited in GC/253, along with other records of the meeting, in archive and manuscripts, Wellcome Library, London.

haemodynamics of a brand new drug called dobutamine.[2] After a sleepless night I decided to stick to my career plan of hepatology rather than haemodynamics, but when back at St Thomas' soon found an excuse to team up with Ron again – performing liver biopsies via the internal jugular and hepatic veins on sick patients with coagulopathies. Ron could never resist a new challenge and we were soon writing up this first experience of the technique outside the US, where it was pioneered.

Indeed my next stop was indeed the USA – on a MRC travelling fellowship to San Diego to research liver function, a BTA. Although I was in a non-clinical post, indeed had no licence to practice there, I was soon being sent up to the ICU to see referrals on behalf of the head of the gastrointestinal division, who was a wonderful researcher but 'a little rusty on the clinical side'.

From San Diego, the next stop was Liverpool to my consultant post in 1980. Cecil Gray was pre-eminent in anaesthesia at this time and Sherwood Jones was doing great things in the ICU at Whiston Hospital.[3] In no time I was invited in to the ICUs of the Royal Liverpool and Broadgreen Hospitals by Tony Gilbertson and Dickie Richardson respectively.[4] I soon realized that the best way to get my liver failure patients admitted to the ICU was to drop everything when an opinion was sought on one of their patients. Liver patients had (and perhaps still do have) a reputation for rarely coming out alive, and so I was careful to give a box of chocolates to those that did survive so they could take it up to the ICU staff when they came back to clinic. The intensivists at the Royal Liverpool Hospital soon realized that I did a safari ward-round of the hospital on Friday evenings starting about 6pm – cursed by generations of housemen and registrars eager to start the weekend carousing – and so this invariably took in the ICU about 9pm.

My involvement in the late 1990s became more cerebral than practical – when I became registrar of the RCP, there were tensions within the intercollegiate training board about the ease or otherwise of physicians getting the requisite training and certification in intensive care medicine – but it was all sorted out amicably in the end with great support from Presidents of the Royal College of Anaesthetists like Peter Hutton and Judith Hulf. Indeed when I was Royal College of Physicians' President, it was a pleasure to work closely with Judith in the establishment of an

---

[2] See page 59.

[3] See pages 4, 24, 25, 48, 51, 52 and 58.

[4] See page 4.

intercollegiate Faculty of Intensive Care Medicine, which will acknowledge the pre-eminence of anaesthesia as a background for entering the specialty but also provide very important access to physician trainees into it too.

This Wellcome Witness account shows brilliantly how multidisciplinary working was crucial; for example, joint working between physician and anaesthetist, Ron Bradley and Margaret Branthwaite or Geoffrey Spencer, in those early days. There is perhaps some truth in Tony Gilbertson's suggestion that support from the rest of the hospital for setting up intensive care units in those early days came easily as other staff were delighted to be relieved of the responsibilities of looking after the most ill patients.

My story of intensive care ran through my personal and professional career and came full circle as my son, training in acute medicine, is now starting a two-year fellowship in intensive care under Professor Richard Griffiths at Whiston Hospital, where Sherwood Jones was so important to the early years of the specialty. I congratulate Professor Tilli Tansey (who became an Honorary Fellow of the RCP during my presidency) and her team on the whole *Wellcome Witnesses* series – so important in capturing what could be so easily lost as the pioneers in various areas of medicine retire and pass away – and this is very much the case with this volume, where the crucial pioneers are now in their seventies and beyond. They should look with great satisfaction on what has been achieved in less than 50 years for the very sickest patients who have entered hospital over this time.

Sir Ian Gilmore
Royal Liverpool Hospital and University of Liverpool

HISTORY OF BRITISH INTENSIVE CARE, c.1950–c.2000

The transcript of a Witness Seminar held by the Wellcome Trust Centre for the History of Medicine at UCL, The Wellcome Trust, on 16 June 2010

Edited by L A Reynolds and E M Tansey

HISTORY OF BRITISH INTENSIVE CARE, c.1950–c.2000

Participants

Ms Sheila Adam
Dr Aileen Adams
Ms Pat Ashworth
Dr Carol Ball
Professor Julian Bion
Professor Ronald Bradley
Dr Margaret Branthwaite
Dr Doreen Browne
Dr Tony Gilbertson
Mr Graham Haynes
Professor Peter Hutton (chair)

Professor Iain Ledingham
Ms Alice Nicholls
Professor Mervyn Singer
Dr Brian Slawson
Dr Geoffrey Spencer
Dr Joseph Stoddart
Professor Leo Strunin
Professor Sir Keith Sykes
Professor Tilli Tansey
Dr David Wright

Among those attending the meeting: Dr Jennifer Jones, Professor Michael Worboys

Apologies include: Dr Richard Beale, Professor David Bennett, Dr Dennis Coppel, Professor Tim Evans, Dr Clifford Franklin, Professor Richard Griffiths, Professor Charles Hinds, Dr Jean Horton, Dr Roop Kishen, Dr Paul Lawler, Dr Robin Macmillan, Dr Willie Macrae, Dr John Nunn, Ms Sue Porter, Dr Alfie Shearer, Dr David Treacher, Professor Nigel Webster, Dr Sheila Willatts

Professor Peter Hutton: Hello everybody. My name is Peter Hutton and I've been asked by Tilli to chair this session, which I'm quite pleased to do, because I think it could be extremely interesting. First of all, some thanks: the first going to David Wright, Tony Gilbertson and Iain Ledingham for suggesting the concept of this meeting and secondly to Tilli Tansey and the Wellcome Trust for receiving the idea so positively and supporting it.

This is a unique opportunity for people to get their word in about how it happened *to them*. This meeting will become part of a series of Witness Seminars, which are written up so that they provide a permanent record of the event. An earlier one on 'Pain Management', for instance, which is relevant to many of us, is extremely good.[1] There are lots of names in there that people will know, and there is an interview with Pat Wall who, of course, sadly died a few years ago. We do want people to speak and we've asked some people to speak on specific topics to get things going from the outset. Once that person has made a few introductory comments, I'm sure a number of people will wish to say something, to add to it from their own experiences.

Start of the specialty (c.1950–c.1960) The 1952 Copenhagen polio epidemic and its consequences The development of equipment and techniques, the conditions treated
Development of units (c.1960–c.1970) Key individuals Key places
Professionalization of staff and their careers (c.1970–c.1980)   e.g. societies; journals; qualifications, training Medical Nursing Technicians
Resources and facilities (c.1980–c.1990) Department, equipment, drugs Record-keeping, scoring systems, transport Other disciplines in intensive care   e.g. Physiotherapy, bacteriology, radiology etc.
Ethics, outreach, high dependency and follow-up (c.1990–c.2000)
Recording the history of British intensive care

Table 1: Outline programme for 'History of British intensive care' Witness Seminar

---

[1] Reynolds L A, Tansey E M. (eds) (2004).

The outline programme on your seats (Table 1) is meant to be flexible; I'll do my best to keep us to time and it's meant to be friendly. So, if I could ask Tony to kick off with the first item, which is to do with the Copenhagen epidemic.

Dr Tony Gilbertson: I was asked originally to speak about the Copenhagen epidemic and I wrote a brief summary, but then I got another e-mail asking me to reflect my views as a medical student during the 1952 Copenhagen epidemic and how, if at all, it affected me then and later as a doctor. I've got to say that in January 1953, when Lassen published his paper in the *Lancet*,[2] I was just about taking second MB and I certainly wasn't reading the *Lancet*, and I didn't read that paper until exactly 40 years later when I was giving a lecture on the history of intensive care at the Royal Society of Medicine, because nobody else had ever talked about it, and I then found out about Lassen and his paper.[3]

But that's not to say that it didn't influence me, because it did. It influenced me indirectly, because Professor Cecil Gray, who was a reader in those days, had actually been teaching in Copenhagen on the World Health Organization anaesthetic course at that time.[4] So he certainly knew all about Bjørn Ibsen.[5] Dickie Richardson ran the intensive care unit (ICU) at Broadgreen Hospital,

---

[2] Dr H C A Lassen (1900–74) was the chief physician at Blegdam Hospital during the 1952 epidemic. His reports on the treatments used include Lassen (1953, 1956); see also Sykes and Bunker (2007): 163. For an examination of the role of Bjørn Ibsen, see Wackers (1994a and b); see also note 7. The two forms of ventilation in long-term use until the 1970s were those administered through a (permanent) tracheostomy or using negative pressure ventilation applied via a tank ventilator, cuirass or jacket/poncho ventilators. Correspondence on the spelling of Blegdam has been deposited in the Wellcome Library, GC/253.

[3] Dr Tony Gilbertson wrote: 'Lassen's name is always given as "Lassen H C A"; his forenames have been very hard to track down, but Sykes and Bunker reveal that he was called Hans Christian Alexander (Sykes and Bunker (2007): 162. Trust Keith to know!' Note on draft transcript, 20 August 2010. See also Gilbertson (1995). Sir Keith Sykes wrote: 'I consulted Dr John Zorab of Bristol who had spent six months working in Copenhagen and who had interviewed one of the young patients treated in the epidemic. John noted that in those days the organisation of the hospital was very hierarchical and most patients would not have dared to question senior medical staff. This particular girl did, however, ask Lassen what his initials stood for. She told John that she remembered that Lassen replied "Hans Christian Alexander" so I included this in the book. Subsequent checking revealed that his names were indeed Henry Cai Alexander as recorded by Wackers (1994a and b). Whether Lassen was trying to make himself seem more approachable or whether the patient's memory was faulty will never be known. Unfortunately the publishers ignored my corrections when recently reprinting the book, so I have not been able to correct the mistake.' Note on draft transcript, 6 March 2011.

[4] See Gray and Halton (1946); see also Sykes and Bunker (2007): 169; Leuwer *et al.* (2008).

[5] Bjorneboe *et al.* (1955).

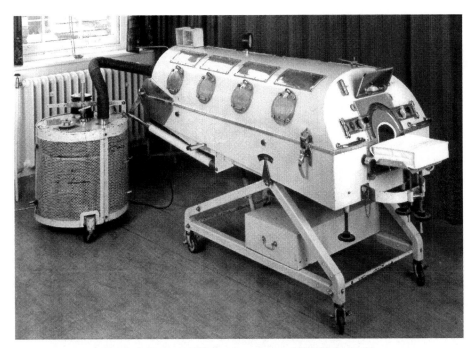

Figure 1: Coventry Alligator iron lung, c. 1966. See note 11.

Liverpool.[6] Actually Pat Ashworth was the head sister so she was running it, but Dick was allowed to have some influence. He'd visited Ibsen in Copenhagen as well. So the influence it had on me was that I realized from a boy that the treatment of respiratory failure was by intermittent positive pressure respiration (IPPR) – sorry Keith, but it was called respiration in those days, not IPPV (intermittent positive pressure ventilation). Up to then treatment had been with iron lungs using negative pressure (see Figure 1), but I realized you had to treat respiratory failure with positive pressure.[7]

---

[6] For the floor plan of the ITU at Broadgreen Hospital, Liverpool, see Figure 7, page 28. See also Ashworth (1964); Edwards *et al.* (1965); Ashworth *et al.* (1973).

[7] Dr Henning Sund Kristensen, an anaesthetist at the department for infectious diseases at Blegdam Hospital from September 1952, disputed the 'principal difference' between ventilation by positive pressure (pressure applied at the entrance of the airways) and negative pressure (pressure created in the alveoli by a total body ventilator or iron lung) (Kristensen (1996): 134). Bulbar paralysis was then considered to be an untreatable neurological destruction affecting the muscles controlling swallowing, talking, movement of the tongue and lips, and sometimes respiration, caused by infection to the 'bulbar' (then comprised of the medulla oblongata, pons and midbrain). Poliomyelitis was later recognized as the cause of this epidemic of obstructed airways and muscular respiratory insufficiency (1994a): 421). For historical details of artificial ventilation and equipment, see Young and Sykes (1990).

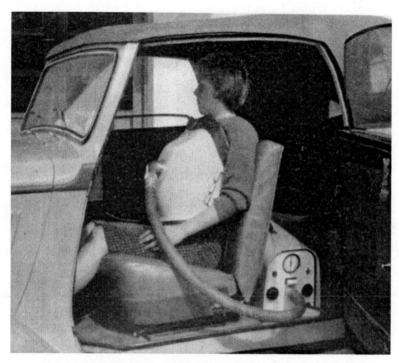

Figure 2: A cuirass shell ventilator connected to a 12-volt alternating suction pump, in use in an Alvis car, c. early 1950s.[8]

I qualified in 1956 and there was no intensive care in Liverpool at that time, but when I went into the Royal Air Force in 1959 I found that the Royal Air Force had embraced Ibsen's views strongly.[9] I say that because we had to bring back patients with respiratory failure, usually due to polio or chest injuries, from all over the world: from the Middle East, the Far East.[10] We had a wonderful system set up by Tony Merrifield and Colin MacLaren, where one of about six of us would get a call: 'You've got to go to Singapore tomorrow and bring back a polio patient.' We'd be met at RAF Lyneham by a technician from the

---

[8] Dr Geoffrey Spencer wrote: 'The Coventry Alligator (Figure 1) was widely used in the UK and other countries and was designed by Captain G R Smith-Clarke, formerly chief engineer/designer to the Alvis Motor Company, Coventry, in 1950. It was made by Cape Engineering Co. of Warwick with money raised mainly by the Coventry Coronation Carnival Committee using a young lady dressed in a long blonde wig who paraded the streets of Coventry on a white horse in 1953.' Note on draft transcript, 2 March 2011.

[9] For problems with transport, see Harries and Lawes (1955). National service (peacetime conscription or call-up) for British men aged 17 to 21 existed between 1949 and 1962, with deferment for education or apprenticeship. See also Royle (1986).

[10] For a recent review of the Copenhagen incident and intensive care medicine, see Wackers (1994a and b).

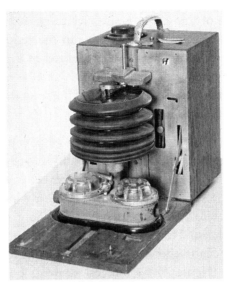

Figure 3: Oxford ventilator: Radcliffe, Mark 1 prototype, c. 1955.
The engine raised the weight and then allowed it to fall and compress the inflating bellows. The inspired gas was delivered to the patient through corrugated tubing connected to a Stott non-rebreathing valve. ©Nuffield department of anaesthetics, Oxford.

medical rehabilitation unit at RAF Chessington where they had the equipment[11] – ventilators and a whole box of equipment – and a sister would come with us. It was very well organized, but I've got to say we hadn't entirely abandoned negative pressure respiration, because I remember bringing an army doctor back from Singapore with polio. He had very much weakened respiration, but no bulbar involvement and I had a cuirass (upper body shell, Figure 2) respirator to bring him back. But the RAF had wonderful Oxford respirators (see Figure 3) with three motors: 12 volts for use in the ambulance; 110 volts for use in the airplanes, which were Comets and Britannias; and 240 volts when we stopped over. Comets were very short-range, so we stopped in Aden or Tripoli. These were wonderful ventilators for the early 1950s with three motors.

To cut a long story short, after learning intensive care in a post-cardiac intensive care unit at Broadgreen, I was appointed a consultant in 1965 at Sefton General Hospital, Liverpool, and for four years I treated patients on the ward without the usual disastrous consequences often described for those treated by IPPV on general wards. What we treated in those days was barbiturate poisoning, asthma,

---

[11] The RAF's medical rehabilitation unit was in Chessington, joined there by the Army's medical rehabilitation unit to become the Joint Services Rehabilitation Unit after 1968. See Ward (1970); for a more recent approach to critical care in the services, see Shirley (2009).

trauma and that sort of thing. But I did have to go in for every staff change of nursing personnel to show them how to run the ventilators. Fortunately I only lived five minutes away. What we specialized in eventually was treating combined respiratory and renal failure, which was because my head nurse, Colette Burrows, had previously been the head nurse on the dialysis unit and so she taught us all to dialyse. The rest is history.[12]

Dr Geoffrey Spencer: I was very interested in what you say about the 1952 polio epidemic in Copenhagen. Dr Henning Sund Kristensen,[13] the anaesthetist who continued to run the Copenhagen unit after the acute epidemic, retired in 1988 and six of the surviving patients living mostly in their homes around Copenhagen transferred their care to me at the Southwestern Hospital in Brixton, part of St Thomas' Hospital, London. One had remained continuously ventilator-dependent via tracheostomy since 1952 and remains so today. She was hand-ventilated (Figure 4) by medical students both during the acute epidemic and for months thereafter until a special ventilator, the 'Pulsula', was developed for her. She found Danish winters too cold and used to spend her winters in Texas until her Texan boyfriend died recently and since then she has spent her winters on the Isle of Wight, evidently the next best thing to Texas.[14]

---

[12] Dr Tony Gilbertson wrote: 'The regional dialysis unit was up the corridor in Sefton General and patients not infrequently developed pneumonia or pulmonary oedema. At first we ventilated them in the dialysis unit but after the ITU was opened in 1970 we dialysed with full support from the dialysis team and reduced the previously very high mortality rate to about 40 per cent. We developed the concept of severe combined acute renal and respiratory failure (SCARRF) and participated in two conferences on the subject in Oxford.' Note on draft transcript, 26 March 2011. See McClelland *et al.* (1990); Gilbertson *et al.* (1991); see also Figure 7, note separate dialysis room. Dr David Morrison's descriptions of the development of dialysis in his intensive care unit in Crumpsall Hospital, Manchester, will be deposited along with other records of the meeting in archives and manuscripts, Wellcome Library, London, at GC/253. See also Blagg (1967).

[13] See note 7; see also Wackers (1994a).

[14] Dr Geoffrey Spencer wrote: 'It is essentially an improved, quieter and better engineered 24-volt modification of the early Oxford Radcliffe machines (see Figure 3) and remains virtually unique. Her ventilator has been adapted to run off aeroplane electrical voltages as well as US mains. This small IPPR machine made specially in Denmark for replacing the medical students was designed by Jø Larsen, medical technician at the Blegdam Hospital in conjunction with two anaesthetists, Dr H S Kristensen and Dr H Poulsen. Larsen made around 50 of these three types – 12-volt, 24-volt and mains for bedside and wheelchair use – which remained in production until 1987. It incorporated a waterbath humidifier and a heated wire inside the single hose to the tracheostomy, which reduced water condensation in the tubing and heated the inspired air. A great pity it was not more widely produced and it probably remains to this day the most suitable IPPR machine for long-term and wheelchair use.' Note on draft transcript, 29 September 2010 and 2 March 2011. See also discussion on page 6; for the personal reminiscence of one of the eight survivors, see Isberg (2005).

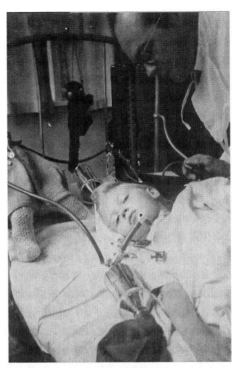

Figure 4: Anne Isberg, aged 8 in 1952, receiving artificial respiration from the black rubber hand-squeezed bag, which the dental student stopped squeezing while the photo was taken, via a Water's canister containing soda lime for CO_2 absorption connected to a cuffed endotracheal tube. The oxygen is supplied from the long tube on the left.

The Copenhagen epidemic was said to have been the first use of tracheostomy and intermittent positive pressure respiration (IPPR, Figure 3) in polio and similar long-term conditions.[15] This is only partly true. Tracheostomy, at least, had been used for so-called 'wet cases' lacking saliva control from the late 1940s in the polio centre at Rancho Los Amigos in Los Angeles, California.[16] They continued, however, to ventilate their patients in an iron lung with a metal collar depressor to keep the tracheostomy outside the iron lung.[17] They did try simultaneously to make this arrangement work better by using a Bennett attachment[18] which gave positive pressure, which worked in synchrony with the iron lung; a startlingly cumbersome system.

---

[15] See note 7.

[16] See www.rancho.org/Rancho_History.aspx (visited 14 March 2011).

[17] See, for example, Baydur et al. (2000); Figure 2.

[18] See Trubuhovich (2007a); and further discussion on page 13.

But to return to Copenhagen, the epidemic has been called 'the 1066 of artificial respiration.' It resulted in the invention of pH, CO_2 and oxygen electrodes by Poul Astrup, a physiological chemist,[19] which made it possible to monitor the adequacy of the medical students' bag-squeezing.[20] It also resulted in the development of the technique and suitable machines for long-term IPPR and patients' eventual home care.[21]

Another point of interest about Copenhagen is 'who asked Ibsen to come?' The people looking after these cases before anaesthetist Bjorn Ibsen appeared were infectious diseases physicians. Professor Lassen's first assistant at Blegdam Hospital was Mogens Bjørneboe – a physician who had worked in the commune hospital in Copenhagen – who suggested to Lassen that the methods of tracheostomy and IPPR might have something to offer. Ibsen came to the hospital and resuscitated a dying girl, one case. Having set her up using a Waters' canister and rubber bag for the medical students to squeeze (see Figure 4), Ibsen left.[22] It is claimed that Ibsen never returned to the polio unit, although the new method was dramatically successful and, with many improvements, still is.[23] Lassen had to be persuaded to include Ibsen's contribution to his 1953 report of the epidemic. But his work was subsequently taken over by a young anaesthetist called Henning Sund Kristensen, who was the person who looked after and maintained the patients until a few years ago.[24]

Hutton: To broaden this a bit, Keith, would you like to say a few words on the development of anaesthetic equipment and techniques at the time?

---

[19] Bjorn Ibsen proposed in 1952 that the death of patients with high total carbon dioxide in their blood at Blegdam Hospital, as measured by manometer, could have been the result of retention of CO_2 from inadequate exchange of air, and that manual positive pressure ventilation could reduce CO_2 levels. Dr Poul Astrup, director of the clinical laboratory, persuaded Radiometer A/S in Copenhagen to develop a smaller pH electrode to measure the acidity of blood, which was delivered the following day. See www.radiometer. co.uk/aceb4403-74fa-4d94-b4a0-6afc24b0b7f5.W5Doc (visited 27 January 2011). For further details of the effects of these measurements, see West (2005), particularly pages 426–8. Correspondence on this point has been deposited in the Wellcome Library, GC/253.

[20] See, for example, West (2005): Figure 3, page 425.

[21] Home care was also important in improving the lives of those on dialysis. See, for example, Crowther *et al.* (eds) (2009).

[22] See Waters (1936); see also Severinghaus *et al.* (1998): S119–20, Figures 4 and 5.

[23] See, for example, Stott (2000); see also note 34. Correspondence on this point has been deposited in the Wellcome Library, GC/253.

[24] See also note 7.

Professor Sir Keith Sykes: An interesting comment about Bjørneboe is that he came back from the US in 1951 on the same ship as Ibsen's wife and family, so that is where the two families got to know each other.[25]

Before launching into the subject under discussion, I would like to thank the Wellcome Trust, not only for funding our history of the Nuffield department of anaesthetics, published in 1987,[26] and for awarding me a number of grants throughout my professional life, but also for being responsible for my entry into intensive care.

It all started one night in December 1958 as a result of a chance meeting with Desmond Laurence outside the Lord Wellington pub (the Jeremy Bentham from 1982) near University College Hospital (UCH), London. Desmond was the clinical reader in pharmacology at UCH and told me that he had just come back from South Africa where he and Barry Adams, professor of medicine in the University of Natal, were running controlled trials on the treatment of tetanus in the King Edward VIII Hospital, Durban.[27] They had been comparing chlorpromazine with the conventional treatment with phenobarbitone and had found no difference in mortality in neonates with severe tetanus.[28] Jokingly I said to him: 'Well, why don't you get an anaesthetist to go out and treat the patients with curare?' And he said: 'Would you like to go?' And I said, 'Yes.' I thought no more about it and some two months later I got a letter from the Wellcome Trust saying they were going to pay my fare out to Durban and were offering me £1000 for equipment. So I went to see Charlie Newman, the dean of the Postgraduate Medical School, who, much to my surprise and delight, offered me six months' leave of absence with full pay. I sold my car to pay for the travelling expenses of my wife and young family and spent six months in 1959 setting up a small respiratory unit to investigate the use of curare and mechanical ventilation in the treatment of adult and neonatal tetanus. Two years later we were able to report a reduction in mortality in neonatal tetanus treated with curare and mechanical ventilation from 84 per cent to 44 per cent.[29] By 1966 the mortality had been reduced to 36 per cent.[30]

---

[25] Further examples of 'Been to America' or BTA, are mentioned on pages 41–2 and 59 and were an important part of the professional development of a number of fields, see, for example, Reynolds and Tansey (eds) (2009); Crowther *et al.* (eds) (2009); see also Sykes (2008).

[26] Beinart (1987).

[27] Laurence *et al.* (1958).

[28] Adams *et al.* (1959).

[29] Wright *et al.* (1961).

[30] Adams *et al.* (1966).

When I returned to Hammersmith Hospital, I found that some of the open-heart surgery patients were dying from what appeared to be respiratory failure, and I made a number of critical remarks about their postoperative treatment. As a result I was asked to join the anaesthetic team and began to initiate treatment with mechanical ventilation after operation. I borrowed the large Radcliffe positive-negative ventilator that Hugh-Jones[31] had used in 1959 to treat asthma and, fortunately, the first few patients survived.[32] We continued to treat the cardiac patients and some patients with tetanus in side wards over the next year and opened a postoperative recovery unit in March 1961. By this time we were treating other conditions such as asthma and acute-on-chronic respiratory failure, so we soon became a general intensive care unit.[33] That is how the Wellcome Trust kick-started intensive care in Durban and in the Hammersmith Hospital, London.[34]

I have been asked to say a few words about what happened before Copenhagen. Polio was rife in the US and, in addition to local infectious diseases hospitals, there were four big polio units using tank ventilators in Los Angeles, Boston, Ann Arbor and Houston.[35] Geoffrey Spencer has already mentioned the groundbreaking papers of Bower and colleagues,[36] in which there were descriptions of some 40 new devices, largely engineered by V Ray Bennett, which improved the care of patients in tank ventilators. As a result this group had managed to increase the survival rate in tank ventilator patients from about

---

[31] Dr Philip Hugh-Jones was on the scientific staff of the MRC Pneumoconiosis Unit, South Wales (1945–55), and later was consulting physician and director of the chest unit at King's College Hospital, London, and part-time director of the MRC Clinical Pulmonary Physiology Research Unit at the Hammersmith Hospital, London (1964–67). Professor Sir Keith Sykes wrote: 'Hugh-Jones was one of the leading respiratory physiologists of the day and, with John West, was responsible for initiating the use of mass spectrometry in respiratory research and the use of radioisotopes for studies of regional ventilation and perfusion in the lung.' Note on draft transcript, 6 March 2011. See Fowler and Hugh-Jones (1957); see also, for example, Hugh-Jones and West (1960).

[32] Russell et al. (1956); Figure 3. See, for example, Gilson and Hugh-Jones (1949); Ness et al. (2002): 31–3.

[33] Professor Sir Keith Sykes wrote: 'We always used to call it acute-on-chronic respiratory failure, since the admission to hospital was precipitated by an acute infection.' Note on draft transcript, 6 March 2011.

[34] Sykes (1964). Professor Sir Keith Sykes wrote: 'Sykes et al. (1969) was the first book to provide a comprehensive plan of treatment for all types of respiratory failure. It was translated into Spanish, Italian and Polish and there were pirated editions in Russia and India.' Note on draft transcript, 6 March 2011.

[35] See, for example, Horstmann (1985).

[36] Bower et al. (1950a and b).

20 per cent in 1946 to over 80 per cent in 1949. This was where Bennett had developed his PR-2 ventilator – the forerunner of many other ventilation devices designed by this brilliant engineer.[37] So that was quite an important development in the intensive care field, and Ibsen was aware of these papers before he was called in to help at Blegdam Infectious Diseases Hospital in August 1952.

I think the shock tents during the war were another important forerunner of intensive care because that's where anaesthetists learnt about triage, about monitoring, about transfusion, and above all, about teamwork. I think we have to realize that there was very little teamwork in medicine before Copenhagen and this development represented a major change in the way doctors interacted with each other. The care of the unconscious patient was also being refined, because Carl Clemmesen, consultant psychiatrist at Bispebjerg Hospital, had started to develop the idea of specialist poison units to treat barbiturate poisoning,[38] and Erik Nilsson had produced his thesis on the benefits to be derived from applying anaesthesia principles to the care of the unconscious patient in these units. At this time, however, there were only a few intermittent positive pressure ventilators and their use was largely restricted to the provision of controlled ventilation during anaesthesia for thoracic surgery.[39]

There was one other interesting antecedent of intensive care and that was a paper in the *Lancet* in 1934 by Howard Florey and his colleagues.[40] They had tried to treat experimental tetanus in rabbits with curare and small tank ventilators without much success, but they made the comment that the best way forward would be to create centralized units, where people with tetanus could be taken to be treated. So in 1934 he and his colleagues anticipated the concept of intensive care. Postoperative recovery wards of course, were, in many cases, the immediate progenitors of intensive care units, but, as Geoffrey Spencer has said, it was the people who went to Copenhagen and started using IPPV instead of tanks (iron lungs) in their fever hospitals who spearheaded

---

[37] In 1956, the Puritan Compressed Gas Corporation acquired V Ray Bennett and Associates, Inc., after Bennett had constructed his first resuscitator unit for a Los Angeles hospital. For further details of the company history, see www.francisfoundation.org/pulmonary.htm (visited 7 September 2010). See also Wilson and Roscoe (1958); Trubuhovich (2007a).

[38] Jensen (1974).

[39] See, for example, Nilsson (1951); see also Sykes and Young (1999): Ch 1, pages 1–19.

[40] Florey *et al.* (1934).

the move to intensive care. Of particular importance were the Oxford group, who established the principles of humidification and other aspects of care that formed the basis of ventilator treatment.[41]

So that is, I think, the background to intensive care. We all know what happened afterwards: Poul Astrup, Ole Siggaard-Andersen, John Severinghaus and others developed apparatus that enabled us to obtain accurate blood gas measurements.[42] The participation of anaesthetists in cardiac surgery and neurosurgery taught us to use other clinical measurements, and during the next two decades we witnessed an explosion of knowledge about the physiological aspects of mechanical ventilation. We then had the description of acute respiratory distress (ARDS) by Ashbaugh and his colleagues in 1967,[43] and the introduction of positive end expiratory pressure. In the same year papers from Nash and Northway and their colleagues alerted us to the problem of high airway pressures and lung damage.[44] Then, in 1971, the introduction of the first microprocessor-controlled ventilator, the Siemens Servo 900, opened up the possibilities of developing new techniques of respiratory support that have culminated in the techniques used today.[45]

Hutton: Julian, I think you were going to add a few points.

Professor Julian Bion: Only in terms of downstream consequences from Bjørneboe. I'm at the University of Birmingham and I come to this later than previous speakers because I was born in 1952. We are now bordering on the brink of the eradication of polio, I'm pleased to see.[46] But thinking of Lassen's paper in the *Lancet*: one of the points that emerges from it is that although

---

[41] See, for example, Marshall and Spalding (1953); Honey *et al.* (1954); Smith *et al.* (1954); Beinart (1987), especially pages 118–23 for the ITU.

[42] See for example, Siggaard-Andersen *et al.* (1960); West (1996): 100–5.

[43] Ashbaugh *et al.* (1967).

[44] Northway *et al.* (1967); Nash *et al.* (1967).

[45] For a background to artificial ventilation equipment, see Young and Sykes (1990); see also Tobin (ed.) (1994).

[46] In 1998, the Global Polio Eradication Initiative (GPEI), supported by UNICEF, the World Health Organization, Rotary International and the US Centers for Disease Control and Prevention, Atlanta, was established to immunize every child against polio until transmission ceased. On 27 January 2011 the US government and the Russian Federation signed a protocol in Geneva to deepen this support. For further details, see www.polioeradication.org/ (visited 3 February 2011).

the mortality rate was reduced from 90 per cent to 40 per cent, of those who died following the introduction of positive pressure ventilation, the time it took them to die was very much longer – from three days up to many weeks – with the new approach. I think that's a theme that will come to inform some of our discussions about rationing and the use of scarce resources.

Gilbertson: My comment was going to be about the long learning curve. It wasn't just a learning curve, as I see it. The delay in instituting intensive care in this country had several reasons and the main one was that Ibsen was said to have opened the doors of the operating theatre for anaesthetists. But talking to people – and I've been interviewing them for the last couple of years – about that time, the point they make strongly is that most anaesthetists didn't want to escape from the theatre. [Laughter] They were what Tom Boulton called 'session anaesthetists' – only in the hospital for a limited number of hours each week – and there was no way that they could look after patients for days on end.[47] Developments of the Health Service in the 1960s increased the number of consultant anaesthetists and gave them competent junior staff so that they could provide continuous care for intensive care units. For instance, there was a 37 per cent increase in the number of consultants – not anaesthetists – between 1952 and 1962, and the Platt report in 1961 had a great deal to do with that.[48] I was appointed as a result of the expansion by the Platt report. I was told by Cecil Gray that if I was ever going to come out of the Royal Air Force, I had better come out now, because they were going to appoint a large number of anaesthetists. In my particular experience, in my hospital, that was absolutely true. After about five of us were appointed in 1964/5, there were no more appointments for 12 years. So I think the ability of anaesthetists to respond to Ibsen was delayed until political change in this country had taken place.

Dr Aileen Adams: I was interested in Keith's comments about tetanus, because this was indirectly why we at Addenbrooke's had one of the earliest intensive

---

[47] A twenty-first century description of a session anaesthetist in hospital policy documents is one who will assess the fitness and suitability for anaesthesia for all patients undergoing general anaesthetic and will be responsible for administering the anaesthetic and associated decisions. See also Boulton (1989, 2007); Boulton and Wilkinson (1995).

[48] Sir Robert Platt's working party recommended that hospital boards should review medical staffing, with advice from consultants, producing proposals for additional consultant appointments and for posts in the medical assistant grade. The report urged the development of the 'firm' system, the reorganization of the consultant service, the development of rotational schemes of training for senior registrars and the establishment of regional advisory committees on senior registrars. Anon. (1961); Ministry of Health, Department of Health for Scotland, Joint Working Party (1961).

care units. We were in an agricultural area, so we had an enormous amount of tetanus. In fact they said up until the vaccination for tetanus came in, that Addenbrooke's was never without at least one case. In the 1930s – 1934 – Leslie Cole, who was the senior physician, took up a suggestion that had been made in about 1811 and 1812 by Benjamin Brodie, the distinguished English surgeon and physiologist, that maybe curare had a place in treating tetanus.[49] That's rather a long time ago, when you think of it. Leslie Cole got some crude, gourd curare and he started to use it in tetanus in the 1930s and published three papers, two in the *BMJ* and one in the *Lancet*.[50] He didn't get very far and was bothered, because, of course, his patients didn't breathe properly. Harold Youngman, who was the senior anaesthetist there, suggested that perhaps he could help, because the anaesthetists were used to dealing with patients such as this. Of course, being a physician, Cole rather pooh-poohed the idea. As you say, he didn't like anaesthetists particularly; they were very low in the hierarchy. But Harold again was unusual; he was quite prepared to spend his whole time in the hospital; he remained a GP anaesthetist and started numerous other things which I haven't time to tell you about, but he kept at it.[51] I think this was one of the reasons – admittedly not until after the war – that we set up an intensive care unit in Cambridge in 1959, which was quite early. Thanks to Harold Youngman as anaesthetist and thanks to a very perceptive matron, Miss Mima Puddicombe, who said she was fed up with nurses not being able to look after patients properly, because they were scattered throughout the hospital.[52] Her own office was converted into an intensive care unit, which was referred to as the Blue Room. Not because the patients were blue, but because the wallpaper was. I think it's interesting that in Cambridge it was tetanus, rather than polio, that was the way into intensive care. I would like to end this by saying this is not my research, it is Jean Horton's research and she wasn't able to be here today.

Professor Mervyn Singer: I'm from University College London – a long way away – that is, across the road. I even post-date Julian, being born in 1958. About a year ago I had to prepare a talk, which prompted me to read the original papers by Lassen, Ibsen, Engström and Astrup regarding the Scandinavian polio epidemics of the early 1950s. For whatever reason, they seemed to target British

---

[49] Brodie (1812).

[50] Cole (1934, 1936, 1938); Cole *et al.* (1968); Cole and Youngman (1969).

[51] See Horton (1992), freely available at: www.histansoc.org.uk/Proceedings_files/Volume_11.pdf (visited 1 September 2010).

[52] Puddicombe (1964).

journals such as the *Lancet* and *BMJ* for publication. There was a wonderful coincidence of people and skills available in Copenhagen at the time. I had the honour of being at Ole Siggaard-Andersen's Festchrift in 1992,[53] and was then told that the reason they got into blood gas monitoring in Copenhagen was because of the presence of Radiometer A/S, Copenhagen,[54] an offshoot of Carlsberg, that developed pH monitoring for the brewing industry. These published papers emphasized the importance of multidisciplinary teamwork and of the crucial role of physiotherapy. They also shot down the romantic view of altruistic medical students bagging the paralysed polio victims by stating they were paid 30 shillings (£1.50) per shift. They made the important point, as did Julian, about the mode of death. A major advantage of blood gas monitoring was the realization that either they were under- or over-ventilating their patients. Over-ventilation caused haemodynamic compromise, so many died from an iatrogenically induced haemodynamic collapse. After recognizing this issue, patients survived, though a further group then suffered later deaths from pneumonia. This was a very interesting shift and was rediscovered some 30 years later.[55]

Dr David Wright: I'm from Edinburgh. I'm going to ask one or two questions, perhaps, rather than giving information. One thing that strikes me is that you need a critical mass to start things off, and in Copenhagen that occurred with the number of people involved in an epidemic. One question is: were there other epidemics that produced that number of people elsewhere? If this was so in Britain, before units were set up, patients must have been managed singly, so which different places were patients ventilated in? Were they side rooms of wards; were they the recovery rooms of operating theatres? But the first question is: were there other epidemics?

Bion: I think there are others more expert than I here. North America is the answer to the first question. The second one would be informed by those who actually looked after the patients and that's not for me to do.

Dr Margaret Branthwaite: This is a slightly flippant comment, and I'm not sure that the word epidemic is correct, but the advent of cardiac surgery had an enormous impact, at least from the mid-1950s onwards.

---

[53] Anon. (1993); see also Burnett (1993).

[54] Radiometer A/S, Copenhagen is a subsidiary of the Danaher Corporation. See www.danaher.com/about/history.htm (visited 27 January 2011).

[55] For further details, see Wackers (1994a and b); West (2005).

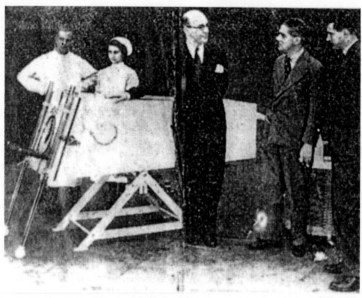

Figure 5: A British iron lung (R to L) flanked by the Australian designer E T Both, next to Lord Nuffield speaking to Robert Macintosh, Nuffield professor of anaesthetics (1938). Macintosh drew Nuffield's attention to the lack of iron lungs in Britain in 1938 and thus Lord Nuffield arranged for production of the machines in the Morris Motors factory in Cowley, Oxford.

Professor Leo Strunin: I was a medical student in Newcastle from 1956 onwards, and there they used to ventilate patients with tetanus by hand. As medical students, we got paid to do it, there was great demand, and you could tell when there was a tetanus patient, because they were ventilated in a side room off one of the wards on the ground floor, and carpets would appear in the corridor to cut down the noise to prevent any seizures. When the carpets appeared, everybody would queue up because one could get paid. [Laughter]

Sykes: There were lots of epidemics of polio that were documented from the late nineteenth century onwards. I think Copenhagen took the record, but polio was endemic in the US and, in 1955 for example, we had a polio epidemic in Boston with some 30 patients nursed in iron lungs in a ward at the Massachusetts General Hospital. There were many other cases treated in the Haynes Memorial Hospital and the children's hospital.[56] Then there was the

---

[56] Professor Sir Keith Sykes wrote: 'There is a graphic description by a patient admitted to the Haynes Memorial Hospital during the 1955 epidemic at: http://emilylee19.com/haynesmemorial_files/ b29cf014ab010ab257abf86752e4e006-0.html (visited 9 March 2011).' Note on draft transcript, 6 March 2011.

1938 epidemic in Britain that precipitated the building of the Both ventilator in Oxford (Figure 5).[57]

So, certainly there were lots of epidemics and the disease was greatly feared by the general population. Most patients in Britain were treated in the special polio units. Macrae in Bristol has written extensively about his unit, which had a number of tanks and later he went on to design and utilize the Clevedon ventilator.[58] But even in Blegdam Hospital in Copenhagen, they only had one tank and six cuirass ventilators, so there weren't many machines around. In the US, however, the National Foundation for Infantile Paralysis had collected enormous sums with its March of Dimes Fund, and you've probably seen the pictures of 40 or 50 tanks in a ward at Rancho Los Alamos Hospital in California.[59]

Certainly in Boston, trying to work in that crowded ward was very difficult. Three anaesthetists went to help out in the ward: Thorkild Waino-Andersen from Denmark, Mike Andrew from the US and myself.[60] We used to have to bronchoscope the patients, but there wasn't enough room because of the tank right behind you. But there was one other thing that was interesting and that was that some of the tanks had a Hoover vacuum cleaner on the top. Every hour an alarm clock mechanism activated the Hoover, which increased the negative pressure in the tank so that lung volume was increased for a minute before returning to normal levels again. That was the influence of Ferris and Pollard who believed that the artificial sigh prevented atelectasis.[61]

Dr Brian Slawson: I'm also from Edinburgh.[62] It's interesting that infection seems to have been the origin of intensive care in some places – in Edinburgh it

---

[57] See, for example, Sykes and Bunker (2007): 181–91; Trubuhovich (2006).

[58] The Clevedon ventilator was designed to treat poliomyelitis by Dr James Macrae and his colleagues at Ham Green Hospital, Bristol, in 1953 and built by Willcocks Engineering Co., Clevedon. See, for example, Macrae *et al.* (1953); see also www.johnpowell.net/pages/clevedon.htm (visited 7 September 2010).

[59] The 'March of Dimes' was an annual fundraising event of the National Foundation for Infantile Paralysis, a US health charity founded in 1938 by President Franklin D Roosevelt, who had been paralysed by the disease. This label superseded the original title of the charity in 1979. See www.marchofdimes.com/mission/history.html (visited 1 February 2011); see also Paul (1971): 88. For a recent review, see Melnick (1996).

[60] Sykes (2008); Sykes and Bunker (2007).

[61] Ferris and Pollard (1960).

[62] Dr Brian Slawson wrote: 'Assisted ventilation was provided in an annexe of the postoperative recovery room of the Western General Hospital from 1966 until the appointment of consultants with sessions in intensive therapy and the provision of purpose-built accommodation there in 1988.' Note on draft transcript, 23 October 2010.

was crush injuries of the chest.[63] Dr Harold Griffiths battled with the surgeons as to what would be the best way to treat them.[64] They wanted to sew the chest together and he wanted to ventilate. He showed that those who were ventilated survived more often than those treated surgically.

The final stimulus to setting up an 'assisted ventilation unit' happened one day when we had to look after a patient with staphylococcal pneumonia and the student ward in the Royal Infirmary was empty for a short time, and the anaesthetists moved in patients and equipment, much to the annoyance of the physician in charge of that ward. The professor of medicine expressed doubts about whether the anaesthetists were fit to have charge of patients.

Professor Iain Ledingham: I'm from Glasgow, Dundee and various other places. Could I follow David Wright's example and ask a question. Keith, with regard to these people performing hand-ventilating of polio patients or supervising, as you described the procedures: what was the risk to those who were looking after the polio victims? Were any records kept of the prevalence of acquired infection among carers?

Sykes: I don't know about that, but after I left Boston in September 1955 I did hear that two doctors and a nurse had gone down with polio in that particular epidemic.[65] So it certainly was a risk and one accepted it, as you did with all those things at that time.

Spencer: Just before we leave the subject of polio, I think we should mention the pioneering work of the Oxford group, who extended the Danish work and developed the simple East-Radcliffe ventilators.[66] This was mostly due to

---

[63] Dr Brian Slawson wrote: 'Patients with tetanus were numerous in other places, such as Leeds and Cambridge. Like them, Edinburgh is surrounded by rich agricultural land, but cases of tetanus were rare.' Note on draft transcript, 23 October 2010.

[64] Griffiths (1960); Bargh *et al.* (1967).

[65] Emergency admissions for polio during the summer of 1955 at the Children's Hospital, Boston, forced doctors to triage patients in their cars. Several staff contracted polio, and two patients had babies while being treated. Later it was discovered that some of the vaccine given in May 1955 to 6- and 7-year-olds in Massachusetts contained live polio virus, which caused some cases of polio. See www.childrenshospital.org/newsroom/Site1339/mainpageS1339P1sublevel132.html (visited 4 February 2011).

[66] Professor Sir Keith Sykes wrote: 'The East-Radcliffe was introduced in 1961 and I adapted this machine so that it could be used as an anaesthesia ventilator as well as in the ITU.' Note on draft transcript, 6 March 2011. Sykes (1962).

the neurologist John Spalding and anaesthetist Alex Crampton Smith[67] – I mention that specifically because Crampton Smith's obituary is published in *The Times* today.[68]

Gilbertson: Very briefly. Trubuhovich – I never know how to pronounce his New Zealand name – says in his review of Ibsen's work that none of the students in Copenhagen got polio. I don't know how he knows, but it's in his paper.[69]

Dr Carol Ball: I'm from the Royal Free Hospital, London. From a nursing perspective, I'm fascinated to find out if anybody knows what the nurses were doing? Mervyn raised the issue of physiotherapists, but did you notice any nurses around looking after patients on cuirass machines or with iron lungs?

Sykes: In Boston there was one nurse to every one or two iron lungs, but I don't remember seeing any physiotherapists. Physiotherapy was something that I learnt from Alex Crampton Smith. I spent some time with Alex in 1957, and he taught me how to remove secretions by manually hyperinflating the lung followed by chest tapping and chest compression on expiration.[70] When we started the unit at Hammersmith, the physiotherapists were extremely supportive and often came in voluntarily at weekends.[71] The nursing staff also helped with the bag-squeezing physiotherapy and suction. It all depended on them. Now I gather that all that lovely tapping and slapping has gone by the board, and you don't do it any more, I made all our registrars do bag-squeezing physiotherapy three times a day, with or without a physio, so that they knew what the lung felt like and could see how the chest moved. I used to think that was the best training that they had because it got them into contact with the patient.

---

[67] See note 41.

[68] Anon. (2010); see also Sykes and Bunker (2007): 79–82.

[69] Professor Preben Berthelsen wrote: 'I have been looking through all the old papers on the polio epidemic. Unfortunately, I can find only one paper – and it is Danish – where it is stated that none of the 1400–1500 students and doctors who ventilated the polio patients contracted the disease (Maag 1953))….I am convinced, however, that the myth is correct. Denmark is a small country. A polio victim among the medical personnel would not have escaped the interest of the medias and would not have been missed by the medical community in a "small provincial town" as Copenhagen was in the 1950s.' E-mail to Dr Ron Trubuhovich, copy to Professor Sir Keith Sykes, 11 March 2011, forwarded to Mrs Lois Reynolds. See, for example, Trubuhovich (2004); see also Trubuhovich (2007a and b).

[70] For the use of physiotherapy in the treatment of cystic fibrosis, see Christie and Tansey (eds) (2004): 5.

[71] See Clement and Hübsch (1968).

Gilbertson: Back to nurses: I gave a lecture about a month or two ago, at the Association of Anaesthetists. It wasn't very well received, because I made the point very strongly that nurses claimed to be the initiating factor – maybe not in intensive care, but certainly in intensive care units – because they were the ones who had to try to nurse people and they didn't feel competent to do it, and they were all over the wards.[72] I actually had to write to the archive of the *Nursing Times* – which is in Edinburgh and they're very good people – and I sent them a list of 24 articles that I'd found written by nurses in the early days of intensive care.[73] In all of them, they claim that they started intensive care units, and I think they make a very good point. I'm trying to raise the status of nurses in the history of intensive care, but the Association of Anaesthetists wasn't the right place to do it. [Laughter]

Dr Joseph Stoddart: This point of nursing: when the Intensive Care Society (ICS) first opened its doors, we had a message from a very senior nurse – I won't say how senior she was – but she said she thought it was incorrect that we should call ourselves 'intensive care', we should call ourselves 'intensive therapy', because nurses always care intensively. [Laughter]

Hutton: Perhaps we should seamlessly slide forward to how intensive care units developed across Britain over the next ten years from 1960 to 1970. Iain, I think you were going to say a few words.

Ledingham: Thanks for inviting me to set the ball rolling on this particular topic. My credentials are that I graduated from Glasgow in 1958, two years post-Tony Gilbertson from Liverpool, and almost immediately found myself involved in both clinical and laboratory work that set the scene for a lifetime in the intensive care world. If time permits I'll add a few words at the end about the related medical influences in Glasgow at that time.

During the early 1970s, as those of us who were around at that time will readily accept, the quality of care of patients, particularly for those with life-threatening illnesses, was rudimentary by comparison with present state-of-the-art practice. I'm thinking of a variety of things, but postoperative monitoring and care, for example, contrasted unfavourably with the quality of care in the

---

[72] See also Lynaugh and Fairman (1992); Crocker (2007). For a US perspective on nursing in the development of the ITU, see Bulander (2010).

[73] See Appendix 5, pages 107–08. Dr Tony Gilbertson wrote: 'The 24 *Nursing Times* articles on intensive care are rearranged in date order to simplify finding them.' Note on draft transcript, 26 March 2011.

operating theatre, as people have touched on already. In the case of unstable patients – here I'm drawing on my own experience, but I guess it's not unique – this amounted to somewhat basic supervision of patients in the anaesthetic anterooms, followed by transfer to the centre of a traditional Nightingale ward. In the case of the Western Infirmary in Glasgow this meant around the coal fire, which was in the middle of the ward, not so very far away from the oxygen cylinders and so on.

Later, medical and surgical wards allowed some of their side rooms to be used intermittently and, again, I have happy memories of pushing Cape-Waine ventilators[74] in and out of lifts and across corridors from one side room to another. Medical staffing throughout this time was a very *ad hoc* arrangement. There was no formalized provision for medical cover. There were exceptions, and one or two of these have already been cited – I think it was one of Tony's papers on the subject that drew our attention to the work of Jolly and Lee in 1957, who were, I believe, among the very first to set up a so-called post-observation surgical ward.[75] In that sense they were, I believe, well ahead of their time.

Increasing awareness of the inadequacy and inefficiency of the care of patients with life-threatening illness led slowly to the development of intensive care units throughout the country. An influential report from the Department of Health in 1962 facilitated this process to some extent.[76] The *Progressive Patient Care* document came out at that time.[77] It encouraged the thought that intensive care was at the sharp end of things, but the report wasn't very specific in detail and merely made recommendations. Staffing arrangements, for example, continued to be non-standardized.[78]

---

[74] For details of the Cape-Waine 'anaesthetic' and Cape ventilators, see Mushin *et al.* (1969).

[75] Jolly and Lee (1957).

[76] Ministry of Health and the Public Health Laboratory Service (1962); Intensive Care Society (2003).

[77] This concept was first described in the US; see, for example: Haldeman (1959). See also Ministry of Health and the Public Health Laboratory Service (1962); Hartley *et al.* (1968). The Central Health Services Council working party minutes, papers, self-care study, reports, intensive care units and action, 1961–67, are held in BD18/2229, MH159/45–48 and MH133/365 at the National Archive, Kew, London. See www.nationalarchives.gov.uk/documentsonline/ (visited 4 February 2011).

[78] Ministry of Health and the Public Health Laboratory Service (1962); Intensive Care Society (2003); see also Hartley *et al.* (1968).

In those days small units were the order of the day. Gordon and Sherwood Jones described the setting up of a four-bed unit in Whiston Hospital, Prescot, Merseyside, and described the evolution of this unit from 1962 through to 1983.[79] Touching on the topic of nursing, the emphasis in the Liverpool paper was heavily on the importance not only of the nursing contribution to intensive patient care, but also of training and specific training programmes were described. Larger units tended to follow, often responding to specific stimuli. One example was the Royal Victoria Hospital in Belfast, where a 12-bed intensive care unit opened in 1970. This was partly in response to the civil disturbance problem that began to present itself at that time. I remember Dennis Coppel telling us at the time that up to a quarter of admissions there resulted from gunshot wounds or blast bomb injuries, so it is easy to see where the stimulus came from in this connection.[80] Mention has already been made about the importance of cardiothoracic and neurosurgical units, and also, to some extent, the respiratory units for tetanus, polio and so on.

Finally, a quick word about my own introduction to intensive care in the early 1960s. This, I think, came principally from two factors: one was that I was an assistant in cardiac surgery at that time and within about 18 months of starting my training in that programme, I was given the responsibility for looking after the cardiac surgical patients post-surgery – the surgeon taking the view that his work began and ended in the operating room, and his junior staff in collaboration with the anaesthetists could do the honours thereafter – an interesting insight into the thinking at the time. The second was my involvement with the MRC hyperbaric oxygen unit in the university department of surgery, Western Infirmary, Glasgow.[81] Some of you will recall that this was a large surgical–medical walk-in facility that was used over something like seven years for management and research of a whole host of acute medical and surgical conditions. While at the end of the day, hyperbaric medicine proved to be disappointing in terms of its effectiveness in medical practice, the experience gave those of us who were involved at that time tremendous insight into the

---

[79] Gordon and Jones (1998a and b); Gordon *et al.* (2000).

[80] Coppel *et al.* (1973); Gray and Coppel (1975).

[81] Professor Iain Ledingham wrote: 'The first director of the MRC hyperbaric oxygen unit was Professor George Smith (1960–62) – thereafter Regius professor of surgery in Aberdeen. I succeeded Professor Smith in 1962 and remained director of the unit until my departure from Glasgow in 1988 to become dean of the Faculty of Medicine and Health Sciences at the United Arab Emirates University.' Note on draft transcript, 11 February 2011. See, for example, Illingworth *et al.* (1961); Ledingham *et al.* (1968).

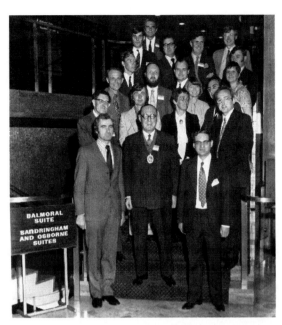

Figure 6: Local organizing committee of the First World Congress on intensive care, London, 1974. L to R: row 1: I McA Ledingham, Lord Brock, A Gilston; row 2: K D Roberts, T J H Clark, G C Hanson, C B Franklin; row 3: M W McNicol, D Williams, J Jones, J Gil-Rodriguez; row 4: A B M Telfer, J C Raison, J B Smith, E B Raftery; top row: J Simpson, E Sherwood Jones, J C Stoddart, D Short, J Mathias.

care of acute illness of all sorts. Individuals who were key collaborators included Bryan Jennett, Ian Donald and Sir David Cuthbertson.[82] Bryan Jennett carried out neurosurgical procedures in the hyperbaric chamber.[83] His team was at the same time developing the Glasgow Coma Scale[84] that became a component of the APACHE (**A**cute **P**hysiology, **A**ge, **C**hronic **H**ealth **E**valuation) critical illness scoring system.[85]

---

[82] Professor Bryan Jennett (1926–2008) contributed to the *Wellcome Witnesses to Twentieth Century Medicine* Witness Seminar on medical ethics education (Reynolds and Tansey (eds) (2007)) and vol. 5 in the series described the work of Professor Ian Donald (1910–87) in obstetric ultrasound (Tansey and Christie (eds) (2000)).

[83] See, for example, Jennett *et al.* (1970); Ledingham (1968).

[84] Teasdale and Jennett (1974).

[85] Knaus *et al.* (1981, 1985). For the background of scoring systems, see Angus (2008): 449, followed by classic papers. Professor William Knaus founded APACHE Medical Systems, Inc. in 1988, the first commercial decision-support software and outcomes management company to disseminate and support the APACHE approach to risk assessment and outcomes evaluation. For further details, see http://hsc.virginia.edu/alive/phs/faculty_page.cfm?id=32 (visited 11 April 2011).

To finish off, at the end of the 1960s a few of us got together and set up the Intensive Care Society.[86] The first challenge we undertook was the First World Congress on Intensive Care, which I think helped to promote the concept of intensive care worldwide (Figure 6).[87] And I like to think that it helped further development of units throughout the UK.

Hutton: Iain, could you comment on Margaret's suggestion that advances in cardiac surgery were one of the stimuli to the setting up of units? Would you agree with that?

Ledingham: Yes, I totally agree with that and it isn't difficult to appreciate why this should be. The concept of tissue oxygen availability and consumption was key to that whole process.[88] So prevention and correction of disturbances in this process were crucial to postoperative care of patients undergoing cardiothoracic surgery. So I very much agree with Margaret's comments.

Stoddart: The way in which the intensive care unit started in the Royal Victoria Infirmary, Newcastle upon Tyne, in the 1950s was because, at that time, Professor E A Pask was the king of all he surveyed.[89] Consequently, if anyone was very ill, or on a ventilator, the duty anaesthetist had to spend the entire 24 hours with him and nothing was allowed to take him away from that. So there had to be a second duty anaesthetist to look after the other patients. Intensive care was very much regarded as being a responsibility of the anaesthetist senior house officer and registrar at that particular time. Everything else developed from there. Pask was certainly responsible for developing the planning of the intensive care unit, which unfortunately

---

[86] For further discussion, see pages 51–2, 56. Dr David Morrison wrote: 'Such intensive care units as there were were largely run by anaesthetists as a part-time hobby. In 1970 Alan Gilston of the National Heart Hospital circulated those of us who he knew had an interest with a view to forming an Intensive Care Society. I attended the inaugural meeting. At that time no-one knew for certain how many units existed in the UK.' Letter on intensive and high dependency care data collection, 4 August 1997. For the aims of the Intensive Care Society, see Appendix 1; for the distribution of the units in England and Wales, see Gilston (1981): 189. The first directory of intensive care units (ICS (1981)) was produced with the assistance of the industrial liaison group, later independently of the ICS (Healthcare Industrial Liaison Group (1987)), along with an annual analysis of ICU statistics. Each ICU received a free yearbook, subsidized by advertising. Letter to Mrs Lois Reynolds from Dr David Morrison, 15 April 2011.

[87] Gilston (1975).

[88] See, for example, Ledingham (1972).

[89] Conacher (2010).

he did not live to see.[90] But intensive care was always something that was regarded from the medical point of view as being the responsibility of the duty anaesthetist.

Hutton: For the folks who were around in that period, was there any central push or planning, or was it local enthusiasms in response to need that made things happen?

Strunin: I worked at the London Hospital (1962–72) and during 1962–65 we were ventilating patients on the wards with uniformly discouraging results. Then Roy Simpson,[91] the professor of anaesthesia, David Ritchie, the professor of surgery, and David Pennington, a consultant physician, presented six of these ventilated cases to a meeting of the medical staff one evening and said: 'This is what's going on in the building. Do you think this is the right way to do it?' Everybody said: 'No.' So Roy Simpson presented a solution. He proposed that the six empty secretaries' offices next to the operating theatres should be used as an 'Intensive Therapy Unit' and he said: 'What we need is to put all the ill and ventilated patients in there, and they will need one nurse each'. At that moment there was a gasp around the room at the concept of one nurse for each patient. I think the final point that made it work, was: 'These beds must be supernumerary to anything else in the hospital', so nobody could just dump a patient in there and forget about them. Therefore, it was agreed, that if whoever was running the unit said the patient was better or worse and shouldn't be there, they went back to their ward. That's what saved it, I think. I believe the unit got going towards the end of 1966.[92]

Ms Pat Ashworth: At the time I was in intensive therapy, I was in Broadgreen Hospital, Liverpool. Intensive care began there when one of the anaesthetists came to the cardiothoracic ward that I was then sister of, and asked: 'How did we feel about our side wards being used for ventilating patients or anything that

---

[90] Dr Joseph Stoddart wrote a protocol for the new 1970 Royal Victoria Infirmary ITU, Newcastle and this was issued to every member of the hospital medical staff: 'The intensive therapy unit provides facilities for the care of patients who require, and would benefit from, more than ordinary ward care. The staffing, space and equipment available enables more detailed observation, recording and treatment than is possible in the busy general wards of the hospital, in which the nursing of the very sick or very dependent patients creates a disproportionate disturbance to the ward routine and to the other patients.' This is reproduced as Appendix A in Stoddart (1975): 188–93.

[91] Dr B Roy Simpson was head of the anaesthetics unit at the London Hospital until 1975 when he moved to Baylor University Hospital, Dallas, Texas (1975–89). See Ramsay (2000).

[92] Mason (1966); Salter (1966).

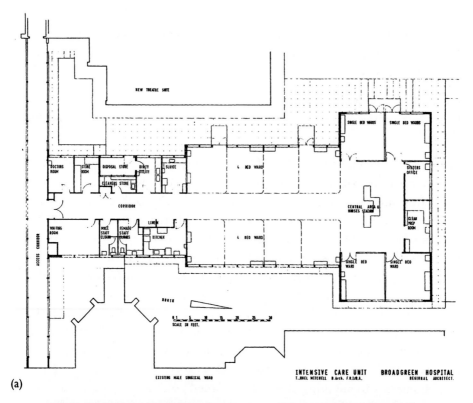

(a)

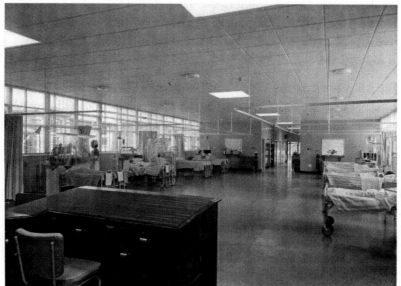

(b)

Figure 7: Broadgreen Hospital Intensive Care Unit, Unit, Liverpool, 1964:
(a) floorplan; (b) view from nurses' station.

needed something beyond ordinary care?' I think we had just combined two wards and been very busy. They decided I thrived on organized chaos. So we said: 'Yes, we would do it.' For the first four years the intensive care unit, not only for the 100 cardiothoracic surgery beds, but also for the rest of the 600-bed hospital, consisted of those two side wards. We had the usual two sisters, myself and a junior sister, and a staff nurse. The remaining staff were all student nurses, so it was quite usual for us to have a couple of patients across the corridor in the side wards flat out, attached to ventilators, students looking after them being end of first year, beginning of second year, while a senior student nurse and junior were in the ward, and whichever of the qualified nurses was on, ran between them dealing with whatever crisis there was.

So it began in a fairly basic way, but on the basis of that experience, I think the primary initiator was the senior surgeon with his other colleagues, who got money from the Nuffield Provincial Hospitals Trust, and some from the Liverpool Regional Hospital Board, and we built the first – it was said by the Ministry of Health nursing officer to be the first purpose-built UK intensive therapy unit (ITU). It was semi-prefab and the 12-bed unit opened in February 1964 (see Figure 7).[93]

That unit was for cardiothoracic patients and then included open-heart surgery, which began in that hospital after we opened the unit. We also had general intensive therapy. The nurses, as I say, had up until that time largely been pre-registration students. At that point we then had more qualified staff, although we always still had three students for their 'experience'. Although we had lectures, I wouldn't call it a course. I refused to call it a course until it could be a proper educational experience. Whereas the hospitals that were running courses very often admitted they were doing it to get staff and the courses were of variable quality and not necessarily a good educational experience. But I would say that we got quite a long way, even in the first four years, learning how to nurse patients who needed ventilation and various other rather extreme forms of treatment. Certainly once we'd opened the 12-bed unit, we had a great deal more experience.

In a way it is quite a surprise to me that so many of the patients survived, despite the fact that they were nursed by inexperienced students with supervision from such qualified nurses as there were. For example, somebody who fell 50 feet in

---

[93] Liverpool Regional Hospital Board, East Liverpool Hospital Management Committee (1964); see also McLachlan (1992).

Cammell Laird's shipyard and ended up with a flail chest, where a segment of the chest wall bones breaks and becomes detached from the rest of the chest wall, and a head injury, went out of the hospital on his feet. Similarly, somebody with multiple injuries with fractured ribs, pelvis, head injury, 'tib and fib' and various other things, also went out on his two feet, eventually.

One of the big problems for nursing was getting the right equipment. In a previous life, I had been running an ear, nose and throat (ENT) ward after the war where we had laryngectomies among other things, and had had to use a mutilated funnel in order to give inhalations to somebody after laryngectomy, because we didn't have tracheostomy masks in those days. By the time we got to intensive therapy, we were beginning to get things like that. But some equipment was still difficult to get. When I visited the US in the mid-1960s, they were using the burettes, which were built-in to the disposable transfusion giving sets, but we couldn't get them in England despite the fact that it was the same firm that was making them.[94] So getting equipment was quite difficult.

Branthwaite: There's one other aspect of circulatory monitoring from that period that I think is worth commenting on, because although a lot of what was done emerged out of the operating theatres, and particularly cardiac surgery, there was also the fact that Ron Bradley at Thomas' in those days was trying to use the techniques of the cardiac catheter lab in the acutely sick and developed his float catheterization technique of the pulmonary artery.[95] It wasn't a question of bringing the patient to the set-up; you took the set-up to the patient. A large trolley was wheeled around the wards (Figure 9), which had the monitoring apparatus, the ECG, the blood gas analysis and so on, and much recording apparatus. Ron and I – I had the privilege of working with him then – were deemed the 'death watch beetles', because unfortunately we weren't always successful. You, Ron, may wish to add to this.

Professor Ronald Bradley: I came to this business from an almost unrecognizably different aspect from all the rest of you. It had virtually nothing to do with ventilators and that end of the business at all. Albeit, in 1956 I was the houseman on the medical unit at Thomas' and we had patients in the open wards, Nightingale wards, on ventilators. People with Guillain–Barré acute infective polyneuritis were ventilated, perfectly successfully, and it worked

---

[94] For a report on clinical experiences of MRC plastic sets manufactured by Capon Heaton & Co. Ltd, see Jenkins *et al.* (1959).

[95] Bradley (1964).

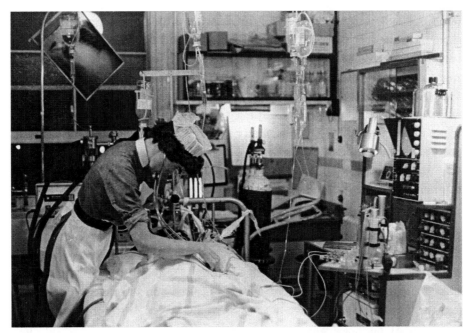

Figure 8: Ron Bradley's equipment in use on a patient after cardiac surgery in St Thomas' north theatre recovery room, c. 1964.

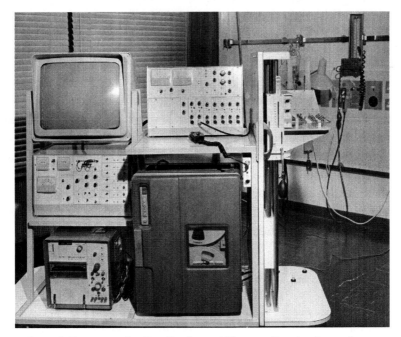

Figure 9: Equipment that Ron Bradley and Margaret Branthwaite used to wheel round St Thomas' before the designated ICU, the Mead ward, was opened in 1966.

alright. That's about all that I had to do with ventilators. I happened to be the HP around at the time. It was later on that I fell into this business of intensive care. What happened was that I spent a number of, not hours, but many days, many months as the medical long-stop at Thomas'. You were called the resident assistant physician (RAP). The day before you were the resident assistant physician, you were an ordinary, ignorant, stupid registrar who was as likely to foul everything up as anybody else. But the day you became the RAP you could hear it around the hospital: 'The RAP says this is such and such.' And that was it. Suddenly you had this sort of god-like touch and it was terrifying. I sat there wondering what the hell they'd show me next.

Now the problem was when I grew up, you could be taught a great deal about chronic medicine, but nobody ever told you how to deal with some acute mess that arrived in casualty and nobody had the foggiest idea what was wrong with the patient. And out of terror, I designed a logic system for myself to sort out these acute messes, so that you could do it with a certain amount of equanimity, and the terror level went down as the system got better. After some time doing this I discovered that it was absolutely useless going and trying to root out help from people like the cardiologists. If you were presented with somebody who was palpably dying of some ghastly sort of circulatory nonsense, if you asked the cardiologist to help, they said: 'Oh, make him better, and then I'll catheterize him'. [Laughter] This was no help at all.

It gradually dawned on me that if only a few straightforward simple measurements could be made, it might be vastly better for this chap when he was very sick, and be more likely to make him better for the cardiologist. Well, Peter Sharpey-Schafer asked me what I was going to do. Schafer had been the professor of medicine and Schafer and Dornhorst were the two halves of the medical unit.[96] They were both remarkable men and very different. And Schafer said: 'What are you going to do?' I replied: 'It's no good if you go to the cardiologist to ask to help you sort out the acute problems that arise. They won't do it. Whereas, with a few measurements, you might be able to do something about it.' Schafer actually rubbed the side of his nose, I remember, and there was a long, long pause. At the end of it he said:

[96] Professor Peter Sharpey-Schafer (1908–63) was professor of medicine in the university unit at St Thomas' Hospital, London (1948–63); see McMichael (1964). Professor Tony Dornhorst (1915–2003) returned to St Thomas' hospital medical school, London, after the war as reader in medicine in 1949 and consultant in 1951, later appointed to the foundation chair of medicine at St George's Hospital Medical School (1959–80). See Collier (2003). For further discussion about this partnership, see Reynolds and Tansey (eds) (2008a): 11; for their contribution to clinical research, see Reynolds and Tansey (eds) (2000).

'Take three years and see what you can do.' So I found myself sawing up lengths of steel tubing and making a scaffolding and putting wheels on the bottom of it so that we could take four pressure heads, a set of gas electrodes and an ECG and a recorder on which you could write the pressure records and everything else that came out. One rather important bit of the kit was a centrifuge so that you could tell what the haematocrit (erythrocyte volume fraction) was doing. All that was on wheels and we went anywhere there was trouble: into the middle of the wards or to the small wards where a lot of these patients were sequestered.[97] I remember sleeping on a sort of terrazzo floor of the old north wing theatres after the cardiac surgeons had done their worst. We looked after those patients overnight with this array of measuring kit. So, I came to intensive care from a very different aspect, which had very little to do with ventilators.

After a time, I think it was about 1966, Geoffrey Spencer presented us with an ideal place in which to work. He built this wonderful intensive care unit that had no walls or very few walls. It was open-plan where you had plenty of space to do almost anything you could think of. It was wonderful. It was a stroke of genius for which I have never thanked him enough, I think. It was a very remarkable place and it became a happy hunting ground for sorting out these circulatory problems. We constructed a system of analyzing mathematically what was going on in the circulation: how was the circulation misbehaving, not only in people with various patterns of coronary artery disease, but also in people with big pulmonary emboli? How was the circulation in people with chronic obstructive airways disease? These people all had different patterns of circulation. Most importantly, people talk of septicaemic circulations as though they were all the same, but they aren't; they're wildly different. Unless you analyse them in this sort of way, you won't do very well for the patients.[98]

The last thing I would like to say is that built into this, there was a gradual development of the kit we used. Most of it was built for us by a marvellous chap called Tony Cowell, an electronics engineer, who built the things on circuit boards. So there was a preamplifier for each of the pressure heads and so on. By that time we'd developed a thermal dilution system for measuring people's cardiac outputs and so on.[99] He put all that onto printed circuit boards and

---

[97] See Figures 8 and 9, page 31.

[98] See Figure 10.

[99] See, for example, Branthwaite and Bradley (1968), which includes an image of Dr Margaret Branthwaite's neck to illustrate the technique for inserting a needle into the internal jugular vein (page 435).

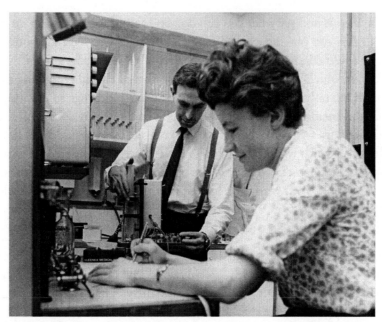

Figure 10: The aftermath of a session investigating cardiac output: Ron Bradley sterilizing the pressure transducers and Margaret Branthwaite 'counting squares'.[100]

when I was chasing him for more and more and more of these things, this man produced out of nowhere, the BBC Micro. This machine offered a measurement system on an incredibly cheap basis. The BBC Micro would provide you with preamplifiers for all the kit, four pressure heads, the cardiac output system, everything. And, it only cost £350.[101] If only the health service had a system somewhere for producing kit for the hospitals, the whole thing could have been done that way. It is still the case that if you go round to the Brompton, and in all of these units, they have separate preamplifiers for doing absolutely everything. Each one costs god knows how much. The opportunity was lost, because I remember the boss of Simonson & Weel Ltd (Sidcup, Kent) in this country coming round and saw this kit based around the BBC microcomputer and said: 'If this is put around and marketed, it will put us all out of business.' We wouldn't be able to afford to send somebody around to all the hospitals to keep

[100] Dr Margaret Branthwaite wrote: 'Thermal dilution curves were originally drawn on graph paper and the only way to determine the area under the curve was to count the squares.' E-mail to Mrs Lois Reynolds, 17 June 2010; Figure 10.

[101] BBC Micro: £235 Model A (16 KB RAM, 1981), £335 Model B (32 KB RAM, 1982) were designed and built by Acorn Computers, Cambridge. Some documents from the BBC Computer Literacy Project, are freely available at: www.bbcdocs.com/joomla/index.php?option=com_content&view=article&id=73&Itemid=69 (visited 31 August 2010).

the kit working if you could buy the machine to do all the processing for £350, and anyone can pirate your programmes.' So, that opportunity is still there, out there somewhere, but it is totally lost now, I think, and it is a great pity.

Ledingham: A quick comment, following on from Leo Strunin's reference to how the unit in his hospital was set up. It reminded me that the way intensive care came about in the Western Infirmary in Glasgow during the period from 1965 through to 1968 was partly as a result of the *Progressive Patient Care* documentation,[102] but also on the initiative of Sir Edward Wayne, Sir Charles Illingworth and Herbert Pinkerton from medicine, surgery and anaesthesia, respectively. These departmental heads got together and decided that the unit would be multidisciplinary from the outset. It has remained so. The great attraction to me, working there for the next 20 years, was that this approach largely addressed the concerns that intensive care was going to take patients away from physicians and surgeons. The referring clinicians had an input to the system and there was a commitment from the start, in terms of both dedicated medical and nursing staff. The unit was seen very much as a baby of the whole hospital, not just an individual department.

Dr Doreen Browne: In 1968 Dr Hilary Howells set up the first three-bedded ITU at the 1000-bedded Royal Free Hospital, London.[103] They didn't have a cardiac surgical unit in those days, nor a neurosurgical ward that involved ventilatory support for their patients. In the beginning it was very difficult, because there was quite a lot of antagonism from clinicians who somehow seemed to view the admission of one of their patients to the unit to be a reflection of failed management on their behalf and so felt resentful. They were always anxious for the patient to be discharged sooner rather than later. The fact that their patient was now being managed by an anaesthetist with their ventilatory expertise was a further cause for concern as they feared loss of control of their patients.

In order to get the unit established at all at the Royal Free, it had to be agreed politically that the patients would remain under the nominal care of the admitting consultant. As time went on, a multidisciplinary unit was established with a major input from the developing renal unit, the liver unit, neurology/ neurosurgical unit, cardiology, haematology, microbiology, chemical pathology and radiology as appropriate, all coordinated by a consultant anaesthetist and a

---

[102] See note 77.

[103] For details of further developments, see Browne *et al.* (1974).

junior anaesthetic team with expertise in modes of ventilation and management of the critically ill patient on a 24-hour basis.

Bion: I have one comment and a question. The comment is that in terms of equipment, we mustn't forget the humble syringe driver, without which we would find things a lot more difficult. My question, which I'd like to direct to Margaret Branthwaite and Ron Bradley – particularly with Mervyn Singer here, who led the PAC-Man study,[104] which demonstrated that pulmonary artery catheters do not appear to improve patient outcomes – is as follows: would you very briefly tell us the story of how the Bradley–Branthwaite catheter became the Swan–Ganz?

Branthwaite: The technique of measuring cardiac output by thermal dilution was reported in rabbits from some time back. We worked it up for use in man using thermisters mounted in the end of Ron Bradley's float catheters.[105] Jeremy Swan, as I understand it, was an Irish cardiologist who had emigrated to the US, and during a return visit to the UK after the thermal dilution technique was in use at St Thomas', he expressed great interest and spent a long time with Ron in the laboratory in Mead ward that Geoffrey Spencer had constructed to his design. Jeremy Swan was full of enthusiasm. As he left, he asked that we should send him the details of the technique. In those days, I was the scribe who typed out in immense detail on a very old manual typewriter with a very grey ribbon, how we made our own thermal dilution catheters. The letter was sent, and as far as I know it was received, but unfortunately it was never acknowledged. It was with some sorrow that shortly afterwards – within a year I think – we saw the publication of a notice of this spectacular new device – the Swan–Ganz catheter – which not only allowed you to measure the pulmonary artery pressure, but also allowed you to calculate and measure the cardiac output as well. Sadly credit was not given where credit was due; that is to Ron.[106] The Swan–Ganz catheter was much greater in diameter than Ron's catheters – which were only half a millimeter internal diameter – and had a balloon. The one disadvantage of the Bradley catheter was that you often couldn't get them through a hugely dilated right ventricle, because they would spin round and couldn't get gripped by the pulmonary artery. On the other hand, they were much less likely to

---

[104] The pulmonary artery catheter (PAC) is also known as the Swan–Ganz catheter (see pages 39–40). For the PAC-Man study, see Harvey *et al.* (2005).

[105] Branthwaite and Bradley (1968).

[106] Ganz *et al.* (1971). For further historical detail, see Swan (1991), one article in an issue devoted to the Swan–Ganz catheter, including a reprint Amin *et al.* (1986a–d); see also Swan (2005).

do any harm, and there was no need to wedge them, because if you had a good undamped pressure trace in the pulmonary artery, unless the pulmonary vascular resistance was enormously high – you could tell from the shape of the curve – you could get the left atrial pressure from the end diastolic. So the Bradley catheters in their original form were, I believe, a very safe device, unlike the Swan–Ganz, which was fatter and had a balloon. They did give us such an enormous amount of information, which I think Ron has already tried to set out.[107] It does seem rather sad that yet another British invention crossed the Atlantic and acquired a different pedigree as a result.

Bradley: Can I chip in a little bit? I'm sorry, but Billy Ganz was a marvellous chap. He got out of Czechoslovakia as the Russian tanks moved in. He thought up this wheeze of putting a balloon on the end of it. It is a remarkable device. It's lovely because the balloon does tend to float the thing in to the place you want to get it; and it does give you a proper left atrial pressure even when you've got a bit of hypertension. It doesn't when you've got severe pulmonary hypertension, but there it is. It was a great device and Billy was a great, good-hearted sort of soul, who I didn't feel did us any injustice at all. No, I have great sympathy with Ganz.

Singer: The question I have for those people working in the 1960s is how knowledge was disseminated? Iain made the point that the Intensive Care Society didn't come into being until the end of that decade. How did practitioners learn what constituted best practice? It seems like intensive care evolved in different areas according to local need, but how did you learn what to do? [**From the audience:** By mistake.] How did you learn from other people? There weren't many review papers, for example.

Mr Graham Haynes: I'm a nurse, not a doctor. I was in Leicester Royal Infirmary in the 1960s. The majority of intensive care patients, or all of intensive care patients, were trauma, particularly flail chest and multiple trauma. I'm going to introduce the awful subject of children in intensive care, because to some it is an anathema to have children in an adult intensive care unit. Children in Leicester Royal Infirmary went to the Children's Hospital. We specialled burns in side cubicles, of which there were a significant number. On the adult general wards we had ventilated patients; asthma and Guillain–Barré syndrome; and on the trauma wards, ventilated patients were also there, a lot of whom would come

---

[107] See Bradley *et al.* (1970, 1971); Jenkins *et al.* (1973).

out of mucky fields because of the surrounding agricultural area. As a student nurse, we learnt by mistake, I regret to say. There was no body of knowledge, in terms of available literature at that time.[108]

Spencer: I cannot let my great ex-colleague Ron Bradley get away with saying that the unit at Thomas' was a work of genius: the only work of genius that I did was to ask Ron and Margaret to come and work in it (Mead ward, Figure 11). [Laughter] I must, however, tell you how the unit came into being, because it was very little of my doing. I came back from working in Shackleton's tetanus unit at Southampton to Thomas' in 1960 and said that Thomas' needed an intensive care unit. I was told very firmly that Thomas' could do anything anywhere and didn't need an intensive care unit. [Laughter] I noticed that Steve Semple, later the professor of medicine at the Middlesex Hospital, and Ron, were treating the acute exacerbation patients with chronic bronchitis by tracheostomy and IPPR in general wards using Smith Clarke volume cycled ventilators and getting into all sorts of difficulties. I tried to help and we published a paper in the *Lancet* describing our results in 29 cases.[109] The mortality was very high from various tracheostomy complications and cross-contamination through the unsterilized ventilators, and including cross-infections to adjacent patients in the medical ward.[110] This reached a point where we were granted two bed spaces for each of these patients, which cost the physicians beds. The cardiac surgeons wanted some special units for their postoperative work and the physicians agreed that an ITU was needed. There was a discussion in the medical committees and everybody said: 'Wonderful idea, but not in my beds.' Fortunately, the hospital was building its first significant rebuild after the war – the east wing – and there was a 28-bedded ward planned to go on the same level as the four operating theatres. The professor of surgery had decided that that ward would be his. I was only a very humble senior registrar at the time, and the hospital administration decided that they could quietly appoint this senior registrar to turn this 28-bedded surgical ward into an intensive care unit (Figures 11and 12).[111] Because it was done under the counter, I had control and

---

[108] Mr Graham Haynes wrote: 'I have been reflecting on the seminar and have been somewhat happy and sad since the experience, which I had not expected. My sadness was personal and coming to terms with my advancing years, but happy that I made a contribution to ITU work through the 1970s–80s and stated so whilst at the meeting. If you did a nursing/ITU seminar, you'd get another perspective and more nurses attending.' E-mail to Mrs Wendy Kutner, 21 June 2010.

[109] Bradley *et al.* (1964).

[110] Phillips and Spencer (1965).

[111] Bell *et al.* (1974).

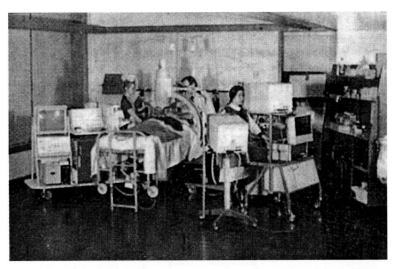

Figure 11: Dr Ron Bradley measuring a patient's cardiac output by thermodilution, assisted by staff nurse Douglas. Valerie Arnold is monitoring the equipment, Mead ward, St Thomas' Hospital, c.1973.

could do more or less what I liked, with a help of the planning nurse, a planner, an architect and a couple of consulting engineers. And that's how it happened. As I said, the only thing that I did that was really useful was to ask Ron and Margaret to come and work there, and to dump their trolley, which was hideously heavy, in the laboratory. [Laughter]

Gilbertson: I'm having a delightful afternoon. I have never met Professor Bradley before, but I'm actually his disciple. I read about his work with plastic tubes being floated in to the pulmonary artery and I bought a drum with a roll of some hundreds of yards of plastic tube – little minute stuff it was – and then I had to try to sterilize it. I spent hours trying to drive the bubbles and the germs out and when I read in the *New England Journal of Medicine* about the Swan–Ganz catheter, I think that was the main reason that I imported some.[112] Was it Seattle that they were in? I rang them up and bought six of them with my own money. After 30 of these catheters had been used, I wrote a paper in the *British Journal of Anaesthesia*.[113] The first citation was Bradley. I'd never met him; I didn't even know where he worked, you know. The London teaching hospitals to a Liverpudlian were these names, there's Guy's and St Thomas' and all the others. I wouldn't even know where to find any of them. But I did acknowledge

---

[112] Swan *et al.* (1970).

[113] Gilbertson (1974).

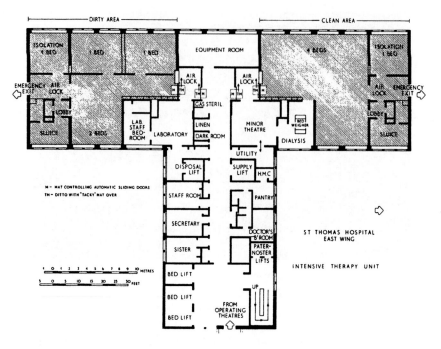

Figure 12: Floor plan of St Thomas' intensive care unit, which opened in September 1966. See note 111.

it. I was very pleased to hear you (Ron Bradley) mention what a nice chap Bill Ganz was, because he and I used to do a double-act, sort of selling these things for US hospital suppliers. He'd tell how he made them and I'd say what you could use them for, and we went all over the place together. I remember giving him some of my *Valium* on a particularly bad flight somewhere. But I've watched with sorrow, in a way, the various reviews that have showed that they were of no use.[114] Certainly not as they were often used, particularly in other countries. I saw one big paper in the American literature about the Swan–Ganz catheter used for prostatectomy.[115] Well, I can't imagine why anybody would want to use the Swan–Ganz catheter for monitoring perfectly healthy people with prostatectomies. We used an awful lot at first, but gradually fewer. The reason we gradually used fewer was that we had learnt by then what to anticipate. We'd learnt about the circulation and particularly the pulmonary circulation. The dangers of them: well, I must say I've seen some terrible tricuspid granulations in post mortems on my patients, but we never burst a pulmonary

---

[114] Pearson *et al.* (1989); Shoemaker (1990).

[115] Garcias *et al.* (1981).

artery.[116] And, we never got one knotted. We got a central venous pressure (CVP) line knotted around a pulmonary artery catheter once – that was very tricky – but I think if you followed the instructions, and it wasn't all that esoteric, they were on the box, just follow the instructions on the box – I think you can learn a great deal from them. But, of course, you can measure cardiac output non-invasively much more easily now and perhaps they've had their day. But at the time, I think they were a great advance. I knew nothing about the left heart pressures; I was great on CVP, but they told me a great deal and I think they were for teaching as much as diagnosis.

Ms Alice Nicholls: I'm a PhD student at the University of Manchester, working on the history of intensive care. I wondered if I could push Mervyn's question a little further and ask about how you learnt from each other in the 1960s? Did you visit each other's units? Did you visit units overseas? Could you say a little more about that?

Strunin: Yes, we did quite a bit of travelling. We also presented papers at the Anaesthetic Research Society, the Surgical Research Society and the Medical Research Society.[117] We went to all of them and presented cases that had occurred in intensive care. I can remember travelling up to Iain Ledingham's unit because we did a bit of hyperbaric oxygen at the time; and we spent most of the meeting trying to find out which was the best restaurant in Glasgow. It was obviously an educational achievement. But we did do a lot of travelling, and people came to visit us, of course. But writing major reviews and things like that was not *de rigueur* in the 1960s. People didn't do it.

Browne: We were very privileged to travel round to other units in the UK, and to go abroad to gain further experience in the 1960s–70s. I was very fortunate in 1970/1 to go to Massachusetts General Hospital, Boston, to work as a research fellow in the respiratory care unit run by Henning Pontoppidan for 18 months.[118]

---

[116] Chun and Ellestad (1971).

[117] Founded as the Anaesthetic Research Group in 1958, see Payne (1988), Nunn (1988); for details of the Surgical Research Society, established in 1954, see Dudley (1976); the papers for the Medical Research Society are part of the collected papers of Sir Thomas Lewis (1881–1945), who founded the society in 1930, and are held in archives and manuscripts, Wellcome Library, London, as PP/LEW/D 'Clinical Research and Medical Research Society'.

[118] See, for example, Pontoppidan *et al.* (1972), one of a three-part 'medical progress' report in the *New England Journal of Medicine*, published as *Acute Respiratory Failure in the Adult* (Boston, MA: Little, Brown and Co.) in 1973.

This was a most enlightening and unforgettable experience, for which I shall be grateful forever. Such leave was allowed at senior registrar level and apart from broadening the mind and obtaining insight into the culture of another country, the 'Been to America' (BTA) label was thought to be a brownie point on your CV for a consultant post in the UK.[119] At the senior registrar level, the BTA was almost obligatory. As an apprentice, would you were on the unit all the time with your patients and learning from people who came in and the various consultants who were involved.[120]

Sykes: At the Hammersmith we had 700 doctors and 700 patients [laughter] and a huge number of visitors. In the cardiac theatre there was always a queue of people looking into the mirror on the operating lamp, or the television screen. However, there were very few people running intensive care units and we all knew each other and visited each other's units. That's how we learned.

Ledingham: I'm pleased that Mervyn raised this topic. It has prompted me to recall that in the early days we soon realized the benefit of having a multidisciplinary approach to intensive care. We had inputs from medicine, surgery, anaesthesia and nursing; and we set up a course, essentially presenting the theory behind certain components of the care within the unit, together with on-the-job training. In the process, I suppose we experienced what is now called 'cross-skilling' as far as our clinical activities were concerned. Obviously we benefited from travel elsewhere, but principally to address the point Mervyn was making, we realized that we had a lot to learn from each other and between disciplines, which tended to bond us together in the process.[121]

---

[119] See pages 11 and 59.

[120] Dr Doreen Browne wrote: 'During my time at the MGH I learnt about a "mobile intensive care service" that provided ventilatory care to patients on the wards outside the respiratory care unit. After I had returned to the Royal Free from Boston in 1971, the three-bedded ITU had to close during the bed-gap period 1973/4 when the new hospital was being built. This meant that the six hospitals in the group were without an established intensive care unit. To overcome this problem three special mobile intensive care unit trolleys were designed to be stationed in the accident and emergency departments in three hospitals in the group. Each trolley was thus immediately available for use in any ward in the three high-demand hospitals and could also be easily transported to any of the remaining hospitals in the group.' Note on draft transcript, 7 March 2011. See Browne *et al.* (1974).

[121] Professor Iain Ledingham wrote: 'As a footnote, prior to creation of the unit, the prospective nursing sister-in-charge was funded to visit the few established units elsewhere in the country and benefit from their early experience. See MacQueen and Kerr (1974).' Note on draft transcript, 13 September 2010. See also discussion from a nursing perspective on page 43; Salter (1966).

Bradley: Going back a step, about the catheters: we ended up virtually not using the things. This was because, as I got older – and idler – and less inclined to involve myself in work at all, I discovered with hands and eyes and ears and stethoscope and a logic system, we could actually avoid putting catheters – you had to have the right atrial pressure and you had to know the systolic and diastolic blood pressure and the heart rate. But that apart, there were physical signs there for the knowing eye which, if you fed a total of six things into a calculator, you could know the strokework produced by the left ventricle and the right ventricle and the pulmonary resistance and the systemic resistance. You could know all these things, and I still carry it round with me in my pocket.[122] And you can do it without too much effort. And it's one of the benefits of getting older and idler.

Ashworth: As regards exchanging knowledge for nursing: one of the things that became important was the meetings at the King's Fund. In 1965 there was a multidisciplinary meeting on the design of intensive care units, held at the King's Fund, with about five or six nurses there. The staff there noticed that we had plenty to talk about and so they offered to let us meet again. We started having meetings twice or sometimes four times a year, for the next few years. Those were very useful meetings, because it brought together usually the sister in charge of each intensive care unit from various parts of the country. When I say the country, I mean the UK, not just England. We talked about all sorts of things, anything from the design of units, equipment, nutrition, other things related to patient care, and things like difficulties of coping with matrons and tutors, and so on, who didn't understand what intensive care was all about. We needed their help, but they needed our help too, and at least one representative of each was invited to the next meeting. Those meetings were very useful. Peggy Nuttall had been a nurse and used to attend.[123] She was excellent at asking pertinent questions to make us clarify what we were talking about and she also wrote up the reports of those meetings. I think it probably happened to other people, but I think I ended up writing at least a couple of articles,[124] because Peggy kept kicking me and saying: 'When do I get it?' So those meetings led to a number of things that I'll mention later, but they were very useful for exchanging information, and some of us did visit each other's units.

---

[122] Bradley (1977).

[123] Ms Peggy Nuttall (1917–2008) was editor of the *Nursing Times* (1959–73). See Dopson (2008).

[124] See, for example, Ashworth (1966); Richardson and Ashworth (1966).

Stoddart: Nobody's yet mentioned the very useful BMA publication from its Planning Group No. 1 in 1967 called 'Intensive Care'.[125] It was very good indeed; chaired by Henry Miller, a very good formative paper. But before we change from ancient history, I might mention that one of the jobs that the duty anaesthetist had to do when he went on duty, was to buy a dozen condoms at the local chemist's shop, because, at that time, tracheostomy tubes tended to be very crude, and we found the best ones were silver tubes with a home-made cuff made from a condom on the outside. These things did tend to burst from time to time, but we always had half a dozen ready for changing over. [Laughter] It was a very good way of keeping the tracheostomy tube clean, because, of course, the inner tube was silver, it was taken out, and it worked as an airtight fit as well.

Wright: I'm interested in anaesthetic textbooks as one way of passing on knowledge. My memory of intensive care textbooks is that there were anaesthetic textbooks with chapters on intensive care. There were excellent cardiovascular and respiratory physiology books, but what was the first textbook in intensive care?

Branthwaite: I'm not sure that I can answer that, but I would hazard a guess that if we restrict ourselves to the UK, it might have been Mark Braimbridge's book on postoperative cardiac intensive care?[126] Very early 1960s, I think, but I'd have to go back to look at the dates.

Hutton: This is all interesting, but we need to try to keep to the outline programme (Table 1). If we move on a bit now from the 1970s to the 1980s, we're going to look at the developments from there.

Professor Tilli Tansey: We haven't really done the 1970s.

Hutton: We haven't done the 1970s as fully as we might have but we must move on. In moving on to different things, if we could slant a little bit more towards the professionalism of staff in their careers. I think a number of people were going to say a few words about this, starting, I think, with Sheila.

Ms Sheila Adam: I'm previously a nurse consultant to critical care and now a head of nursing. I'm a little surprised to be asked to do this but I will say something in terms of professionalization. I started as a student in intensive care in 1981 and at that time there was a Joint Board of Clinical Nursing Studies (JBCNS)

---

[125] BMA, Planning Unit (1967).

[126] See, for example, Braimbridge (1965); Fleming and Braimbridge (1974).

course,[127] which – I'm looking at Carol Ball to see if she also undertook that?[128] For the first time nursing had an accredited intensive care course. I'm interested in Professor Ledingham's comments about his course, because I'd be surprised if that was accredited at that time? No? So, it was an internal course only. Very early on, in the mid-1970s and early 1980s, there were clear courses that nurses had to undertake and the course was accredited by, I think, the JBCNS at that time.[129] Moving on from that, we also had an association of nurses that met in London and this was the London Intensive Care Nurses Group. This was designed to improve understanding and share knowledge across the country, not just in London itself when I joined it, and was led by a lady called Patsy Barrie-Shevlin. She took this forward with sheer force of personality, as much as anything else.

Haynes: Could I comment on that please? I undertook my intensive care course at Westminster Hospital – 1972 – and we had an inspection. Pat Ashworth was on that inspection panel. It was nine months long and we had to do a further three months to gain our hospital certificate. We weren't allowed a JBCNS certificate at that time, and I can't remember when that commenced, but I'm sure Pat can fill us in there.[130] There was an informal group of London intensive care-oriented nurses who began a group called the Nursing Intensive Care Group (NICG) London, and this started in 1975. The key people who started that were Pat McCann from the London Hospital; Sue Porter from the Middlesex; Penny Irwin from St Thomas' Hospital; we always tried to persuade the late Jemma Boase to join us, but she was reluctant, Jane Cant from St Thomas' Hospital, plus myself. We were sponsored by Portex and they were absolutely wonderful in the early days of us setting up the group.[131] The London group (NICG) became more nationally oriented and groups set up throughout the country. Eventually we held national conferences based in London. We

---

[127] The Joint Board for England and Wales was established in 1970 under the chairmanship of Sir Hedley Atkins, with representatives from the nurses', midwives' and medical Royal Colleges, the Central Health Department, and the health authorities to ensure a national standard in post-basic clinical education and training for nurses. See note 141.

[128] See page 47.

[129] See note 143.

[130] The curriculum was approved in 1972 and the first certificate was awarded in 1973. See Orme (1985).

[131] Portex supplied plastic tubes for intubation and for ventilation and has been a registered trademark used for surgical and medical apparatus and instruments since 1947, owned by Smiths Medical ASD, Inc., Keene, New Hampshire. See also pages 46 and 59; Healthcare Industrial Liaison Group (1987).

usually had about 400–500 attendees. That group eventually became the British Association of Critical Care Nurses (BACCN).[132]

The push to start a nursing intensive care group came about because of Virginia Henderson, who was the keynote speaker at the Royal Festival Hall for the American Association of Critical-Care Nurses. The American nurses like to hold a foreign jamboree once every five years.[133] From that NICG, we began a journal called *Intensive Care Nursing* and the editorial panel were as stated: Sue Porter, Penny Irwin and myself, and later Nora Flannigan (Charing Cross).[134] Sally Nethercott from Great Ormond Street represented the children's faction. Again, Portex were very helpful. Going back to the literature: when I undertook my course in 1972, there was no recommended reading, and Foyle's on a Saturday morning became the hunting ground for us all, which was quite an undertaking knowing the Foyle's referencing system.[135] We used a Meltzer handbook for coronary care; Braimbridge for cardiac nursing care – it was post-surgery. We didn't have anything at that time for renal, as I remember.[136] For general intensive care there was a US text that came from the Beth Israel Deaconess Medical Center, Boston, Massachusetts,[137] and there was a cardiac and general intensive care book from Green Lane Hospital in Auckland, New Zealand. Those are the ones that stick in my mind.

Ball: Graham has covered quite a lot of the content I was going to mention, but – I'm not sure why as Graham was a contributor – he omitted what became the bible for intensive care nurses in the 1980s, which was the publication by Jack Tinker and Sue Porter from the Middlesex Hospital, London, called *Intensive Care Nursing*.[138] My course at Guy's in 1978 was a JBCNS course,

---

[132] The Nursing Intensive Care Group (London) was established in 1977, with the regional affiliation dropped two years later. In 1982, it was decided a national group was needed and the inaugural meeting of the BACCN was held in 1985, supporting 15 regions. Its journal was first published in 1985, later known as *Intensive and Critical Care Nursing* from vol. 8 (March 1992). See Healthcare Industrial Liaison Group (1987) and www.baccn.org.uk/about/background.asp (visited 30 November 2010).

[133] Mr Graham Haynes wrote: 'Patsy Barrie-Shevlin represented the UK at the New Orleans conference in the late 1970s.' Note on draft transcript, 10 February 2011.

[134] Haynes (1983).

[135] Hoge (1999).

[136] See, for example, Meltzer *et al.* (1965); Braimbridge (1972); see also Appendix 2, pages 91–102.

[137] Pontoppidan *et al.* (1973).

[138] Tinker and Porter (1980).

JBC N100 its number. When I started teaching in 1985, Tinker and Porter was the bible – everybody had to have one. For some years it continued to be so, I would say.

Ashworth: I'm about to talk about the foundations that went behind all that. The meeting at the King's Fund that I talked about continued until 1968; the group of nurses went on meeting, usually about 20 odd of us. Then it became obvious, because we were sometimes talking about things like salary and conditions and work, the King's Fund couldn't accommodate that sort of meeting. It was becoming obvious anyway that we needed to widen the meeting to include more people. Rather than starting an independent association, the decision was that we would go into the college, the Royal College of Nursing (RCN). At that time about 30 per cent of nurses belonged to a professional organization of some sort, and the College was much the biggest. The advantage of going into the College was that we would have a much bigger voice in what we wanted to say about intensive care nursing – if we could convince the officers and the council – than if we were an independent association. Indeed, that was what happened.

Somebody mentioned the BMA report on intensive therapy from the medical point of view;[139] there was also a report from the Royal College of Nursing in 1969, which was written by several of the people, plus others, who had been in this group at the King's Fund.[140] When the JBCNS was set up in 1970, a survey found that there were 350 courses of various sorts in 47 different specialties, and decided that some rationalization was needed.[141] 'Intensive Care Adults' was one of the first four topics where they set up a panel in order to devise a new course. When the first group of us came together, there was a JBCNS clinical nursing studies officer, another nurse educator, and seven other nurses, and six medics, including people like Dr Sherwood Jones and Dr Eric Gardner. Our

---

[139] BMA, Planning Unit (1967).

[140] Royal College of Nursing (1969).

[141] As a result of the 1966 report on the post-certificate training and education of nurses by a subcommittee of the Standing Nursing Advisory Committee of the Central Health Services Council (Powell (1966)), the Joint Board for England and Wales was established in 1970 to endorse a national standard in post-basic clinical education and training for nurses. The background to two reports (Joint Board of Clinical Nursing Studies (1972, 1975)) is described by the Board's principal officer (Gardener (1977)). The Joint Board was dissolved in 1983 by the Nurses, Midwives and Health Visitors Act 1979, and its papers are held as DY1 and DY2 in the National Archives; see www.nationalarchives.gov.uk/catalogue/displaycataloguedetails.asp?CATID=95&CATLN=1&accessmethod=5&j=1#index (visited 22 February 2011). For an evaluation of hospital nursing administration, see Dewar (1978). See also notes 127 and 143.

first task was to ask: 'What is intensive care?', because all the units that we have talked about were different and we had to decide what general intensive care involved; what would we put into this course? As recommended, we devised the five major objectives and the required 'skills, knowledge and attitudes' that went under those. As Graham Haynes mentioned, the first course outline for JBCNS 100 contained a required reading list.[142] Yes, the system was that when the first courses had been approved in 1972, the first intensive care courses were approved by a JBCNS nursing officer, who usually had worked with the hospital designing the course, plus a nurse and a doctor from the specialty. This was one thing that was very different from the usual way nursing course initiation happened; these courses were written almost entirely by clinicians and they were expected also to be approved by clinicians. We went on to design a course for enrolled nurses as well as one for registered nurses, and then for specialist areas like children, renal care and coronary care, etc. In 1979 when the UK Central Council for Nursing, Midwifery and Health Visiting (UKCC) was being set up, it was said that those courses became the English National Board (ENB) courses. In Scotland there was a similar organization that also authorized courses. The important thing was that these developments took place at national level and were nationally approved. Previous to that, the certificates issued from hospitals were only as good as the reputation of the hospital they came from.[143]

I'd like to go a bit further on professionalization, because the question of education remains.[144] One of the things the Joint Board recognized was that many clinicians were teaching on Joint Board courses, but did not have training

---

[142] See Joint Board of Clinical Nursing Studies (c. 1974). A selection from the five objectives for skills, knowledge and attitudes appear in Appendix 2, pages 91–102.

[143] A committee (Committee of Nursing (1972)), chaired by Professor Asa Briggs, was set up in 1970 to advise on the quality and nature of nurse training and recommended replacing the existing nine separate bodies for the UK with a unified central council and separate boards in each of the four countries with specific responsibility to improve standards of training and professional conduct, which eventually formed the basis of the Nurses, Midwives and Health Visitors Act 1979. In 1983, the UKCC replaced the Joint Boards (see note 141). Dissolved in 2002, its functions were transferred to a new Nursing and Midwifery Council (NMC). The English National Board was also abolished and its quality assurance function went to the NMC. For the background to nursing structure, see www.nmc-uk.org/About-us/ The-history-of-nursing-and-midwifery-regulation/ (visited 30 November 2010); Gardener (1977). See also notes 127 and 141.

[144] See, for example, Atkinson (1987, 1990).

on 'how to teach'. This applied both to medics and nurses. First of all the JBCNS did two one-week courses, which were multidisciplinary. The first one, I think, was held at the Royal College of Physicians so the doctors would go. [Laughter] Unfortunately, the regional people did not take up this idea and continue it, so after the first two, the courses were held just for nurses in various parts of the country. These were to help people identify teaching opportunities within the unit; how to identify what could be taught; to look at not only the actual teaching and methods of teaching, but also the assessment that went with it. I think this was an important step forward.

It was very interesting on the first course when, as I say, it was multidisciplinary, because I think I'm right in saying that all the nurses knew that we had a lot to learn about teaching. Quite a number of the medics thought they'd been teaching for years and knew all about it. But we all realized that we had things to learn. As regards societies, as I say, we went into the College. As regards journals: what happened with the first peer-reviewed intensive care nursing journal in this country was that the publisher Churchill Livingstone came to me and asked: 'Did I think there was a need for an intensive care journal?' I replied, 'Yes', because we didn't have a decent level clinical journal at all at that time. We had the *Nursing Mirror* and the *Nursing Times,* which were mainly news journals. I referred them to Penny Irwin at St Thomas' and to somebody else who'd done a supplement with a drug company, but they went to the *Nursing Mirror* to produce a regular supplement. Churchill Livingstone came back and said, 'Do you still think we need it?' I said, 'Yes, because that's only ever going to be a supplement.' So they asked would I please do it? Well, I wasn't actually looking for things to do, but I said that I would, provided that they would let me form a board of people who were still engaged in intensive care, which I wasn't at that time, although I was still teaching periodically. The first issue of the journal came out in April 1985, and it began as *Intensive Care Nursing* and moved on later to be *Intensive and Critical Care Nursing.* I think it was important to a lot of the early courses, because it was the only journal that had material from this country that was particularly relevant. Much that came to us for publication had been written for course assignments and so on. One has to recognize that most nurses at this time, even nurse tutors, had not been taught to write referenced material. They hadn't even been taught to read it. So this was quite a step forward, and initially one had to do a lot more editing. Of course, I had never been taught to do these things, but I learnt over the years. The journal was quite important as a means of exchanging knowledge, both for this country and for other countries, because other than that there were only

US journals, and there were nurses in other countries who needed somewhere to publish things too. I think all of this contributed to the professionalization of nursing. Even in 1974 I was writing about clinical nurse consultants, although not specifically for intensive care. Unfortunately it took us a lot longer than that before we actually had them.[145]

Bion: May I give a brief personal perspective on professionalism and training? I trained as a cardiologist and went into anaesthesia in 1981 because I wanted to do intensive care, and it was the only route. At the time, as others have reflected, the training was very centre-dependent. I have great pleasure in sitting next to my mentor, Iain Ledingham, who established in Glasgow a training centre of clinical and research excellence, but there was no national curriculum for intensive care medicine. That was one of the ways one accessed appropriate training. But, we've moved on from there with the establishment of the Intercollegiate Board, led substantially by individuals who are here now.

Since then we have established a national training programme through the work of the Intercollegiate Board for Training in Intensive Care Medicine with a competency-based training programme, which allows us to integrate across specialties, across disciplines and across geographical borders. So the training programme, in which I was privileged to play a significant part, allows us to compare and share competencies with, for example, intensive care nurses.[146] Of course, the nurses were ahead of us in developing competency-based training. We then took that a step further in the development of the CoBaTrICE programme, the **C**ompetency **Ba**sed **Tr**aining programme in **I**ntensive **C**are Medicine for **E**urope, which has been endorsed by 44 countries worldwide, and fully adopted by ten European countries, one of which is the UK.[147] The CoBaTrICE programme is also shared with advanced nurse practitioners in intensive care. With nurses, we have a blurring of professions, a sharing of skills, and an increasing emphasis on collaborative decision-making.[148]

---

[145] Ms Pat Ashworth wrote: 'Officially 1999 in the NHS.' Note on draft transcript, 8 September 2010. See Audit Commission (1999).

[146] Inter-Faculty Collegiate Liaison Group on Intensive Therapy (1985, 1986); Stoddart (1994).

[147] The CoBaTrICE Steering Committee Partners project was led by Professor Julian Bion; see www.cobatrice.org/Data/ModuleGestionDeContenu/PagesGenerees/en/01-about/0A-collaboration/2.asp (visited 30 November 2010).

[148] For a background to specialist nursing, see Scott (1998).

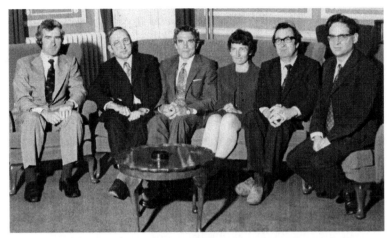

Figure 13: The first council meeting of the Intensive Care Society in 1973.
L to R: Iain Ledingham, chairman; Clifford Franklin; Eric Sherwood Jones;
Gillian Hanson, Joe Stoddart, Alan Gilston, hon. secretary and treasurer.
Dr Keith Roberts is missing from the photograph.

Finally, this year (2010) we have established the new Faculty of Intensive Care Medicine (FICM), formed by seven Trustee Royal Colleges, and housed at the Royal College of Anaesthetists. The FICM has been tasked by the GMC with creating intensive care medicine as a primary specialty programme, by March 2011. We will do this, while retaining the capacity for dual certification between intensive care medicine and other primary specialties. This puts our future on a very secure foundation.[149]

Hutton: What about the Intensive Care Society itself? How did that get going?

Ledingham: The ICS started – well, let us say that correspondence began to be generated around 1969 – and I think all of us who were involved in that correspondence would like to pay tribute to the late Alan Gilston, who was a major force in terms of setting up the Society in 1970.[150] The people who served

[149] The Faculty's trustees are the Royal College of Anaesthetists, College of Emergency Medicine, Royal Colleges of Physicians of Edinburgh and of London, Royal College of Physicians and Surgeons of Glasgow and the Royal College of Surgeons of Edinburgh and of England. The primary specialty training programme for intensive care medicine will run in parallel with dual certification from the FICM and another base specialty. Professor Julian Bion is the Faculty's foundation dean. For further details, see www.rcoa.ac.uk/index.asp?PageID=1523 and www.ficm.ac.uk/ (visited 8 February 2011). For a flavour of the background to the creation of the specialty, see Stoddart (1986); Ledingham (1987); Morgan (1987).

[150] For Gilston's draft structure of the ICS, see Appendix 1, pages 91–102; see also note 86 and Gilston's biographical note on page 139. For Gilston's contribution to early British heart transplant surgery, see Tansey and Reynolds (eds) (1999); see also Ross (1975–77).

on the first council – Joe will correct me if I miss anybody – were Cliff Franklin, anaesthetist from Manchester; Eric Sherwood Jones, physician from Liverpool; the late Gillian Hanson, physician from London; Joe Stoddart, anaesthetist from Newcastle; Keith Roberts, cardiac surgeon from Birmingham; Alan Gilston, anaesthetist from London; and myself, at that time clinical physiologist from Glasgow (Figure 13).

I had the honour of serving as the first president with Alan Gilston as secretary (Figure 14). Harping back to my earlier comments about the Glasgow multidisciplinary approach, the first input to the Intensive Care Society was very much multidisciplinary and, if I remember correctly, this philosophy was built into the stated aims of the society and the hope was that this would continue to be the case for British intensive care.

At that time I already had concerns about the difference in approach between the UK Intensive Care Society and the Society of Critical Care Medicine (SCCM) in the US, which was formed two years later. The SCCM was truly multidisciplinary in the sense that separate disciplinary/specialty chapters (e.g. surgery, internal medicine, anaesthesia, nursing, etc.) were involved from the beginning. This was not the case in the UK Intensive Care Society.

As I said in my introductory remarks, the First World Congress in 1974 was the major challenge for the small group of us who were in at the beginning and we were astonished at the way the arrangements for the Congress developed and flourished over the period of a few months before June 1974.[151] We were amazed (and almost caught off balance) at discovering that around 2000 people would be attending the Congress. We had originally planned for 400–500. At a late stage our professional organizer (Miss Robin Cridland) had to hire a second venue (the Royal Garden Hotel), a not inconsiderable achievement in central London. But to cut a long story short, the Congress proved to be a great success and a tribute to Alan Gilston for having provided the necessary *vis a tergo*.[152]

---

[151] Gilston (1975).

[152] Professor Iain Ledingham wrote: 'Great credit was also due to the many individuals and organizations who overcame immense difficulties at a time of national upheaval in the UK (not least being the three-day working week!). One anecdote, in retrospect brings a wry smile to my face, related to the international scientific advisory committee having to terminate its deliberations in the Royal Society of Medicine at 3pm because that was the time when the heating and lighting were turned off.' Note on draft transcript, 13 September 2010. See also Figure 14 and Appendix 1, pages 87–90.

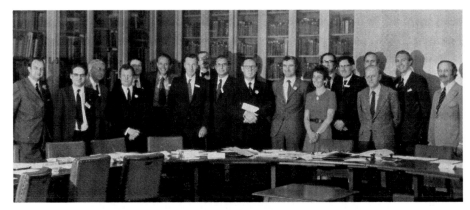

Figure 14: Meeting of the International Scientific Committee of the
First World Congress at the Royal Society of Medicine, 26 June 1973.

L to R: J C A Raison, A Gilston, R Nedey (France), A Milhaud (France),
A Chapman (France), M W McNicol, G Vourc'h (France), A Richard (France),
M Goulon (France), Lord Brock, I M Ledingham (chair),
G Hanson, J C Stoddart, K Roberts, K Peter (West Germany),
H Lutz (West Germany), A B M Telfer, M H Weil (US).

Wright: May I ask how sessions for consultants developed? People were anaesthetists, but then at some stage, people became intensivists. That was not the word that was used, perhaps, at that point, but can I ask how consultants got more sessions in intensive care and who were the first British specialists in intensive care, because this must have been happening during that period.

Gilbertson: I've no idea who the first British specialists were. The phrase *soi disant* would come to mind. We didn't call ourselves that then. But I had no sessions for intensive care for about the first ten years that I was running an intensive care unit and putting in a huge amount of time. When the Royal Liverpool University Hospital was opened in 1979, we were given new contracts and I made jolly sure my contract was for anaesthesia and intensive care. That's when I became a part-time intensivist.

Hutton: It was alluded to the other week in an obituary that Jack Tinker was the first full-time intensivist.[153]

Branthwaite: The question at issue is who was the first full-time intensive care clinician. I would have said, surely, it was Ron Bradley, because he had only

---

[153] These claims in Jack Tinker's obituary (Fricker (2010)) were disputed by Caroline Richmond (*BMJ*, online rapid response, available at: www.bmj.com/content/340/bmj.c2920.full/reply#bmj_el_237308 (visited 13 December 2010)).

been involved in intensive care and had no physicianly responsibilities outside that unit.[154] OK, he was part of a group with others who brought in anaesthetic expertise, but I think in terms of a contract, it would have been as a consultant physician. It's too long ago to remember, perhaps, but it was certainly designated in terms of its intensive care responsibility. And I happened to be senior registrar in intensive care at the same time.

Haynes: In the early 1970s Julian Leigh was a full-time consultant at Westminster Hospital.[155]

Stoddart: Yes. When I came back from the RAF, I was first assistant, and the job of first assistant was to do intensive care. So when I got my consultant job it was an intensive care job with anaesthesia; that way round. I had one anaesthetist session and the rest was intensive care. [**From the audience:** Date please.] 1967.

Ledingham: When the purpose-built unit was opened in the Western Infirmary in Glasgow in 1968, three of us were appointed with sessions in intensive care medicine, surgery and anaesthesia.[156] Since I had by then given up doing surgical lists, for all practical purposes I was certainly a full-time intensive care consultant from 1968 through to 1988.

Hutton: I think we're gently moving on to resources and facilities. You mentioned to me that we haven't said too much about the role of technicians in the development of intensive care, and perhaps we'll return to that shortly. But on this particular section, I think we'd ask that Julian say a few words to introduce the discussion.

Bion: I will reflect briefly on resources, rationing and, perhaps, a bit on scoring. To take a personal perspective, my first training in ICM was in Wexham Park Hospital (Slough, Berkshire), where the ICU had four beds. I was the general medical SHO, the sole medical opinion resident in the hospital. I also

---

[154] Dr Margaret Branthwaite wrote: 'Professor Bradley was initially a research fellow in the medical unit, dealing only with the acutely ill and was appointed a consultant about the mid-1960s, probably when the ICU (Mead ward) opened. His paper on float catheterization of the pulmonary artery is dated 1964.' Note on draft transcript, 19 August 2010. See note 105. See also Sir Keith Sykes' biographical note on page 140.

[155] Dr Julian Leigh was senior lecturer and honorary consultant anaesthesiologist in the Magill department of anaesthetics, Westminster Hospital, London, in 1974, and by 1979 was consultant anaesthesiologist, Royal Surrey County Hospital, South Western Surrey Health District and honorary reader in the department of human biology at the University of Surrey, Guildford. He was Hunterian professor at the Royal College of Surgeons in 1972. See, for example, Leigh (1974).

[156] MacQueen and Kerr (1974): 157–8.

looked after the ICU. It was a disconcerting experience, particularly for the patients. [Laughter] When I became a consultant and senior lecturer in 1987, I graduated to a six-bedroomed 'broom cupboard' at the Queen Elizabeth Hospital in Birmingham, the university teaching hospital. It was routine to have quite significant arguments between the external consultant users – mainly the surgeons – about who should have access to the one available bed. In 1990 we were able to move to a ten-bedded Nightingale ward, which was donated to intensive care by the professor of surgery. At that time it was in the 'gift' of doctors to control use of clinical space. There were five consultants practising intensive care, in addition to the base specialty of anaesthesia. From 2000 until this year, through a process of co-location and expansion, we have developed five ICUs in four geographical locations across two hospitals with about 65 critical care beds. Today, 16 June 2010, my colleagues are starting the process of moving two of those ICUs into the new hospital ICU in Birmingham, where we have a 100-bedded intensive care unit in one single location.

The change in staff is equally remarkable: we now have 32 ICU consultants, which is not enough, and a range of junior staff. Several of the consultants, myself included, practise intensive care medicine full time. We also have intensive care colleagues who have dual certification in respiratory, emergency and acute medicine as well as anaesthesia. One of the new challenges confronting us is how we maintain teamworking and collaboration in such a large critical care area, when there are so many changes of staff because of limited working hours. It is no longer acceptable or legal for trainees to work more than 48 hours, and consequently they work in shifts, which mean that continuity rests solely with the consultant working one week at a time.

While this transformation has been remarkable, and brings with it some new challenges, the issue of rationing has not disappeared. It was when I was working with Iain Ledingham in Glasgow that Bill Knaus published his seminal article on the APACHE II score.[157] We had had privileged information from Bill Knaus about his scoring system and modified it for auditing inter-hospital transfers. When we sent our article to the *BMJ* for review and it was accepted, one of the reviewers wanted to know whether it could be used to deny access to patients who were too sick to require intensive care. That was a fairly obvious question and it has remained a very difficult one to answer ever since. I think we've become much more sophisticated in our understanding now about how

---

[157] Knaus *et al.* (1985); note 225.

to use scoring systems, realizing that they cannot be a substitute for informed medical judgement.[158]

Hutton: I'm sure there'll be things to come. Tilli, just for the record, one of the points we do need to make is that in almost all centres in the UK, there has been a gradual rise in the number of ICU beds. There has been a successful increase – if you can call it that – in the beddage and the recognition of the fact that intensive care units are now an integral part of a modern hospital.[159]

Bion: The expansion in intensive care facilities has come about through a number of key initiatives. The Intensive Care Society has been a consistent advocate for improving resources for critically ill patients. The multiprofessional consensus statement supported by the Department of Health and chaired by Dr Val Day, *Comprehensive Critical Care*, in 2000, was absolutely fundamental in determining the subsequent development of intensive care and de-politicizing this very difficult issue of non-clinical transfers and rationing.[160] We were very much supported in that enterprise by the establishment of the Intensive Care National Audit and Research Centre (ICNARC), whose scientific director is Professor Kathy Rowan.[161] It is through the development of this high-quality case mix programme that we've been able to demonstrate the need for and the appropriate use of, intensive care resources with the publication, which came out in the *BMJ* earlier this year.[162]

Adams: Could I make a couple of points? Firstly, I can remember when people used to be horrified when we were trying to go up to 18 beds. And now I'm horrified that you're going up to 100 beds. What I wanted to say particularly is that there is a transition, and I think it is around year 2000 when we were asked to refer to 'critical care' rather than 'intensive care'. This is important from the number of beds point of view, because we started talking about critical care beds, which included high dependency beds as well as intensive care beds. From

---

[158] See also note 230.

[159] Hutchings *et al.* (2009).

[160] Department of Health, National service framework expert group (2000); note 161.

[161] The ICNARC was created as a result of the UK APACHE II study (Knaus *et al.* (1985), see note 85). In 1991, Dr Kathy Rowan, on behalf of the Intensive Care Society (ICS), submitted a proposal for a national centre for comparative audit and research in intensive care to the Department of Health and received two years' funding. This charity was established as a separate sister organization to the ICS in 1994. See www.icnarc.org/CMS/DisplayContent.aspx?root=ABOUT&AspxAutoDetectCookieSupport=1 (visited 30 November 2010).

[162] Hutchings *et al.* (2009).

then on, the rise in bed capacity hasn't only been about intensive care beds, it's been about high dependency beds or level-two beds, as we used to call them in critical care.

Ledingham: A quick comment, picking up the point that Julian made about patient transfer and leading onto the concept of regional intensive care. For the historical record, I would like to acknowledge the support that we received in Glasgow from the Nuffield Foundation, which funded the first 'critical shock study group' that subsequently became known as the 'shock team'.[163] Shortly thereafter Tenovus-Scotland funded the first mobile intensive care unit in the country, a purpose-built and equipped ambulance.[164] This was the forerunner to what later became the regionalization of intensive care, in our case the west of Scotland. It was a highly exciting programme and, as I say, initially funded by the Nuffield Foundation, and subsequently by the Greater Glasgow Health Board (GGHB).[165] Interestingly, when I was about to leave Glasgow in 1988, the concern was that the shock team would disappear with me. The resultant outcry from the regional hospitals served by the system gave voice to the desire that this should not happen. The GGHB responded positively and, in collaboration with neighbouring boards, ensured the continuation of the regional intensive care service to the west of Scotland.

Gilbertson: Two small points: we've spoken about multidisciplinary work and I'm interested in multispecialty. The unit that I started and ran for years was very much an anaesthetic unit. That wasn't because we were guarding our boundaries, but the physicians have changed a great deal since 1960. When we moved into the Royal Liverpool University Hospital, amalgamating about five small 300–400-bedded teaching hospitals, in 1979 and for a few years afterwards, the most senior opinion for medical patients at night, or outside the consultants' ward days, was an SHO. Even the registrars were resistant to it; they certainly didn't live in. A senior registrar visit was something of a papal visit. [Laughter] Physicians, in my experience, didn't want to have to put in the sort of out-of-hours work that the anaesthetists were doing. I know it's changed now, and it's marvellous that it has. I think it's largely because physicians, and

---

[163] Ledingham *et al.* (1974).

[164] Waddell *et al.* (1975); Ledingham (1978).

[165] Professor Iain Ledingham wrote: 'The contribution of the shock team was recognized in 1986 with the BUPA medical foundation doctor of the year award. The BUPA adjudication panel based their decision on the published work of the group, particularly Bion *et al.* (1985).' Notes on draft transcript, 11 February and 14 April 2011.

even surgeons, are being trained in intensive care or critical care medicine with anaesthetists and so there is a generation of physicians that have grown up to expect to have that sort of commitment. But I'm saying this about physicians, where just up the road from me in Whiston was Eric Sherwood Jones. But he was very much an exception. When the Intensive Care Society was set up, it had a number of physicians; a minimum ratio of physicians to anaesthetists, and as far as I know, had quite a difficulty in recruiting enough physicians at the time.

Stoddart: One thing that has not been mentioned is the importance of pre-planning. We were very lucky in Newcastle, because when the plan for the new intensive care unit was being developed, the chairman was Dr J A G Horton, an anaesthetist, although there were other respectful non-anaesthetist members of the staff on the committee. This chairman actually wrote a planning document to describe what the intensive care unit was for, how patients would get in, how they would get out, who would look after them, who would be responsible for them, who would be responsible for passing on information, what limits (or no limits) were for certain things. The most important part of this planning document was that the ICU was multidisciplinary from the beginning, from the senior house officer staff point of view. Every anaesthetist, every surgeon, every physician who was on the internal rotation in our hospital, spent a time in the intensive care unit: the physicians spent four months; the anaesthetists spent six weeks twice a year; and the surgeons spent four weeks. I think it may have been partly a reflection from that, but intensive care has never been able to attract very many surgeons. That may or may not be a good thing, but the fact remains. This document still exists and is still a very useful document.[166] It tells people who don't quite know what sort of things you can look after in the intensive care unit; how to get them in and how to get them out.

Slawson: I'd like to suggest that the ready availability of very senior help in other specialties other than anaesthesia is partly a result of the changes in training that have taken place following European Union laws.[167] My wife and I have both fairly recently been treated by very senior clinicians at odd times; they were present within the hospital. This is because of changes in the training of the junior staff and consultants are now always present.

---

[166] For the protocol for the Royal Victoria Infirmary's 1970 ICU along with the floor plan, see Stoddart (1975): 188–93, Appendices A and B.

[167] For EU Working Time Directive (2003/88/EC), see http://eur-lex.europa.eu/LexUriServ/LexUriServ. do?uri=CELEX:32003L0088:EN:HTML (visited 24 February 2011).

Wright: We've jumped forward a little bit and perhaps we could go back to the mid-1980s. One of the things that struck me is that we talked earlier about BTA – Been To America.[168] I wondered what people thought about the influence of Australia in the 1980s, because quite a number of my younger colleagues went to Australia rather than to America, and Australia, ahead of Britain, introduced specialist fellowship exams.[169] I wondered what people thought about that?

Browne: The current trend for people to go to Australia would be equally as stimulating as the US, with the added benefit of the chance to obtain the specialist diploma in intensive care medicine.[170] I think that the Australian training – Been To Australia as opposed to America – would be absolutely invaluable. The Australians were multidisciplinary and they had that specialist training diploma years ahead of us in the UK.

Bion: We regard the Australian training as extremely high quality. One of the key things they have done is to establish a collaborative critical care trials group, and they've done that following on from Canada, and we in the UK are now doing the same thing.

Hutton: I think that some of the distances in Australia also stimulated the intensive care of transporting patients, especially when people have to be sent over great distances.[171]

Wright: Another thing from my training in intensive care in that period, or my exposure to learning in intensive care, was the Brussels reunion meetings, where Jean-Louis Vincent and others played a major role in education.[172] The other thing was the role of drug companies in funding such meetings. Lilly, who produced dobutamine,[173] I think, were major funders of the specialty at that point. We've already mentioned Portex being supportive, and I wondered

---

[168] For other discussions on 'BTA', see notes 25 and 119.

[169] Joint Faculty of Intensive Care Medicine, Australian and New Zealand College of Anaesthetists and the Royal Australasian College of Physicians (2003). For further details, see http://ama.com.au/node/3142 (visited 4 February 2011).

[170] For the professional training arrangements in Australasia, see Stoddart (1986).

[171] A Witness Seminar meeting on 'The history of rural medicine and rural medical education' that addresses some of these issues was held on 29 January 2010 and is scheduled for publication in 2012.

[172] See, for example, Vincent and Singer (2010).

[173] A sympathomimetic cardiac stimulant used to treat heart failure and cardiogenic shock; see Tuttle and Mills (1975).

whether anyone else has any examples of industry in the 1980s, or earlier, supporting intensive care?

Branthwaite: Upjohn was certainly one of the notable supporters, partly because they were trying to get *Solu-Medrone* used more widely.[174] It was very controversial at the time, and since. But they supported an annual visit from somebody from this country from an intensive care background to visit a variety of centres in Australasia. I had the privilege of doing this once, but I think that I learned more than I was able to contribute.[175]

Ashworth: As far as nursing was concerned, it may be appropriate to point out that it used to be extremely difficult to get money from drug companies and equipment companies. One of the medics, who had tried to help the nurses to get money for some project, admittedly it was about 20 years ago, was astonished at how difficult it was. I don't know whether that has changed, but I think it is something to be recognized if nurses have been a bit slower to do some of these things.

Bion: To bring the discussion forwards in time, there is a significant change in attitude over the last five years where there's become a much greater recognition of the adverse consequences of too cosy a relationship with industry. The medical profession has acquired an extreme dependence on easy funding from industry. We're in the process of trying to unravel this relationship in such a way that we can maintain the best scientific components of it without having our judgement conflicted too significantly. The other point, perhaps, is the difficulty one has with scientific research funded by industry when it comes to adverse outcomes. I think we can all imagine such examples, which I won't go through now.

Stoddart: A keen supporter of intensive care in the 1970s and 1980s was the British Council, because they paid for me to go to several places and they also paid for doctors to come to work in my department from other parts of the world.[176] I don't know whether they're still doing this on any level, but they were certainly very generous at that time.

---

[174] Methylprednisolone, a synthetic steroid, is injected intramuscularly when rapid action against inflammation is required.

[175] See also note 131.

[176] Dr Carol Ball wrote: 'The director of nurse education at University College Hospital was contacted by the British Council to identify staff trained in intensive care, who were also qualified teachers, to undertake this work.' Note on draft transcript, 3 March 2011.

Ball: I would like to add to that that I also had experience of going abroad for six months with the British Council to Bangladesh in 1987 for education and training purposes. I concur that we nurses were also included.

Wright: Yes, I had a year in Canada during which at least my airfares were paid by the British Council.

Hutton: To stick to some of the topics that we were meant to cover, there is the issue of record-keeping in intensive care as well. It was felt to be an important aspect, I think, by a number of people in the development of the subject. Do people have comments on that, because I think it has changed considerably over the years.

Strunin: I'll make a comment. Again, it goes back to the unit at the London Hospital. We decided very early on that the people who were looking after the patients were the nurses, and so there were limits charts for each patient on whatever things were deemed to be relevant, and within those limits the nurses could do anything they wished. If the situation went outside the limits, the nurses had to call for medical help. The other interesting thing that arose was that the senior nursing ladies, who had nothing to do with intensive care, hated this system, because the nurses were now doing things, such as giving drugs, etc., and they raised the issue of what would happen if a nurse gave the wrong dose or the wrong drug? We invited the Medical Defence Union to come to visit us. The chap had never been in an intensive care unit before and he looked around and said: 'Who are these patients?' We said, 'Well, they're the illest patients in the hospital.' He said, 'Will they all survive?' And we said, 'Well, probably not, you know. The mortality here is quite high.' 'Oh,' he said: 'Then it doesn't matter; nobody's going to find out if you give the wrong dose'. [Laughter]

Member of the audience: I don't think he would say that today.

Ledingham: On this business of record-keeping, and embracing to some extent the next item on that same list, scoring systems. I imagine if I mention the word 'etomidate',[177] it will probably be easy for those present here today to understand how these issues came together. In the ITU at the Western Infirmary, Glasgow, we kept careful records of all the patients from 1975, including the clinical details right through to outcome in individual cases. Before APACHE came into existence there were other scoring systems, which

---

[177] Etomidate (*Hypnomidate*, Janssen Pharmaceutical Ltd, Marlow, UK) is a carboxylated imidazole derivative, a short-acting hypnotic anaesthetic agent developed for intravenous administration in humans.

included the trauma score, injury severity score and so on.[178] The existence of these detailed records made it possible for us to identify a sudden and substantial increase in mortality among our trauma patients in the period around 1982/3.[179] In this audience there is probably no need to go into further detail about this sad story, other than to say that we were extremely grateful that we had kept these detailed records.[180] When we tracked the injury severity scores over the next two or three years, having dropped etomidate from the programme, the mortality returned to what it had been before, as our subsequent publications showed.[181] The pharmaceutical company involved with etomidate gave me and my colleagues an extraordinarily hard time and, as Julian has mentioned, the adverse criticism of our observations was not limited to pharmaceutical companies, but enough said on that score. We do need to emphasize the importance of defining rather carefully the relationship that we have with pharmaceutical companies.[182]

Bion: May I take up an associated theme? To encapsulate it quickly, it is called 'utilization shift'. We see this with the shift from caring for victims of polio to those with the acute respiratory distress syndrome (ARDS), from etomidate in the anaesthetic room to etomidate in long-term infusions in the intensive care unit causing profound adrenocortical suppression,[183] and dobutamine and pulmonary artery catheters to improve outcomes for high-risk surgical patients preoperatively, to the same interventions causing harm in critically ill

---

[178] See, for example, Gunning and Rowan (1999).

[179] Ledingham and Watt (1983). The company (Janssen) agreed to cease promoting etomidate for sedation in intensive care. See note 182.

[180] Professor Ian Ledingham wrote: 'There was extensive correspondence in the *Lancet* following our letter (see note 179). Debate on this controversial issue continued until relatively recently; current evidence indicates that the use of etomidate in critically ill patients should be considered with extreme caution. An excellent review is Cuthbertson *et al.* (2009).' Note on draft transcript, 11 February 2011.

[181] Watt and Ledingham (1984); see also Watt *et al.* (1984).

[182] Professor Iain Ledingham wrote: 'I would like to take the opportunity to acknowledge the support of Sir Abraham Goldberg, then chairman of the Committee on Safety of Medicines (CSM). I well remember being summoned by Sir Abraham to meet with him in his room and being grilled in detail about the evidence for the content of our letter to the *Lancet*. The interview seemed interminable, but the upshot was the circulation of a "Dear Doctor" letter from CSM advising caution in the use of etomidate in intensive care patients.' Note on draft transcript, 11 February 2011. The letter from Sir Abraham Goldberg was dated 20 June 1983 (Anon. (1983)).

[183] Ledingham *et al.* (1983).

patients with sepsis.[184] We've become at last much more sophisticated in our understanding that the population to whom we apply these interventions are very different animals from those where they were first evaluated.

Ashworth: To go back for a moment to the question of the nurses giving drugs: I think a number of situations arose about the question of not just giving intravenous drugs, but things like defibrillation, intubation, various things like that.[185] A number of us who were senior were not against them doing these things, but we believed that it was very important that if nurses were to do these things, it should be agreed policy that they were doing that; they should be properly taught and checked to see that they were able to do it competently; and that it would be acknowledged practice that they could continue to do that. We've been fortunate in the UK that the law does not give a list of things that nurses can and can't do. In countries where they have had those conditions, it is a great problem because it's always out of date. It is necessary for nurses to realize that they are responsible for what they do as qualified nurses, irrespective of what the doctor says. Therefore it was important that if nurses were to do things that they had not been doing previously, that it was agreed policy and they were properly taught and approved as competent.

Adams: I wanted to go back to record-keeping and pay tribute to the large all-encompassing patient chart. It may sound like a trivial thing compared to all the equipment etc., but I think it made a huge difference to really understanding what was going on with the patient where you had your total patient physiology out there in front of you and you could really see what was happening and why.

Singer: I was also going to make a plug for computerized systems. Julian mentioned ICNARC which, apart from being an incredibly useful political

---

[184] Hayes *et al.* (1994).

[185] Professor David Morrison wrote: 'The big breakthrough in the field of cardiology was the development of an effective DC defibrillator by Bernard Lown in about 1953. Prior to this, defibrillation had been attempted with AC shocks, which were rarely effective. Once one could do something about ventricular fibrillation, there was some point in continuous ECG monitoring. Oscilloscopic continuous monitoring had been technically feasible for some years, but few machines were available and were mainly used for research. After Lown, coronary care units were set up and ECG monitoring became commonplace. The electrocardiogram is still the most useful thing to monitor continuously, since it allows one to watch cells at work and gives early warning of severe disturbance of cell function.' From 'Development of ICUs', document written in response to a letter from a nursing officer doing a research project in ICU history, 1992. Original document will be deposited along with other records of the meeting in archives and manuscripts, Wellcome Library, London, held at GC/253.

tool to embarrass government into providing more funding for critical care, has given us a wonderful insight into the epidemiology of intensive care in the UK.[186] Some 90 per cent of ICUs in England, Northern Ireland and Wales – but not Scotland who do their own thing – actually pay ICNARC to give them their data. The database now has over 700 000 patients.[187] The other aspect where we as a specialty have led the way is in the uptake of computerized monitoring, which far outpaces anywhere else in the hospital system. Perhaps this is because we like toys, technology, gadgets. Many units are now completely paperless. This helps to minimize drug error as you don't have to read a doctor's bad handwriting and can instead prescribe using a template.

Hutton: Sorry, when I said 'not everybody is', it wasn't because I don't think computerized monitoring isn't a good thing, it's just a fact.

Bion: There are different levels of evolution, but as a specialty I think, you know, we should pat ourselves on the back.

Strunin: I was going to make a comment about the large paper charts. You're absolutely right, while you've got the patient there, the chart is useful, everyone can have a look at it. But, of course, it is irretrievable data, because once the patient leaves, what are you going to do with it? We had filing cabinets marching down the corridor filled with charts. It is a fire hazard, that's all [Laughter], so you might as well throw the charts away. But when you say you're going to dispose of them: 'Oh, you can't throw them away!' What are you going to do with them? I think the computerized records are obviously the way forward. The difficulty is that there is not a standard system anywhere, as far as I know. We're back to the early days of word processing where everybody did something differently. I've been retired a little while now, but as part of my sins, I used to go round to hospitals to visit intensive care units for the Royal College of Anaesthetists, and I would go to a unit where it is all wonderful and ask: 'How long would it take a new person, a nurse or a doctor, to learn how to use this system?' Sometimes it was weeks, and that raises the question of whether this is

---

[186] See note 161.

[187] Dr David Morrison wrote: 'Every unit I had visited was collecting statistical information for its own use. The basic datasets were similar, although they differed in some respects due to differences in local interest. Most units kept the data in a unit book. This was usually an HMSO book, which the nurses would rule out in biro into columns for the data, a fairly time consuming task….The information collected by nurses and doctors was likely to be accurate, because they would be collecting for their own interest.' Letter to NHS Executive, Department of Health, 4 August 1997, on intensive and high dependency care data collection. See also King's Fund Panel (1989); note 86.

the best way forward. It's something that will have to be tackled and done, but there is a little way to go, I suspect.

Gilbertson: Mixing two things together: we were talking earlier about how people communicated in the early days, in the 1960s. We used the Luton and Dunstable big chart[188] in Liverpool for ages, and every intensive care unit in Liverpool had a chart that said Luton and Dunstable on the top. [Laughter] I got the chart paper from Luton and Dunstable. We did have a lot of communication in those days between the various regions, down the phone, I suppose. The question about letting nurses give dangerous drugs: this leads into something wider as well. The matron in Sefton General Hospital said: 'Well, the nurses can give dangerous drugs, but on two conditions: one is you have to have a morning course to teach them what to give and what not to give and so on, and you give each of them a certificate signed by you; and second, you must write a letter to me saying that you take responsibility for anything that goes wrong.' Matron carried that letter for a long time. [Laughter] So you see, we got on very well. The matrons supported us. But also, one of the things I've noticed in talking to so many people recently for research into this subject is a distinction between, to put it kindly, the teaching hospitals – without particularly mentioning a region – and the problems that my colleagues had establishing intensive care there, because of the competition from people who didn't want their empires disturbed. On the other hand, those of my colleagues who set up intensive care in regional hospitals, the poorer the better – most of them were old work houses – where we were welcomed. When I went to Sefton General Hospital in 1966 we had three regional units: a dialysis unit,[189] a poisoning unit and a medical cardiac unit. I treated patients on the ward for a while, and they weren't doing too badly. But after four years, the physician superintendent came to me and said: 'You're causing disruption on the wards. The tropical people aren't using a ward; would you like a ward for yourself?' I couldn't have had more cooperation. There was absolutely no antagonism, no empire building, no defence of boundaries. And I have noticed that in the teaching hospitals there is a difference in philosophy: 'You're not treating my patients.' Nobody said: 'You can't treat my patients'. They said: 'I think this patient's going to die unless you do something about it.'

---

[188] Ms Pat Ashworth wrote: 'Almost every ICU in Liverpool had a Luton and Dunstable chart, since we had designed and started using our own at Broadgreen by 1964 (though having been discussed and agreed mainly with the cardiothoracic staff, it probably did not suit those working in units that only had general intensive care rather than our mixed patient population).' Note on draft transcript, 7 September 2010.

[189] See note 21, page 10.

And, for a while I walked six feet above the ground, because I thought: 'What a privilege to be able to treat the worst patients in the hospital.' Then I realized that was because the physicians and surgeons wanted to go home. [Laughter]

Adam: I wanted to talk a bit about our attitude change to risk and safety in intensive care, because I think that came about at the end of the 1990s to the beginning of the 2000s.[190] It is my personal impression that we were quite cavalier about what we did initially. We would try new types of interventions – I'm looking here at Mervyn from memories of early haemofiltration and early extracorporeal membrane oxygenation (ECMO) or extracorporeal carbon dioxide removal (ECCO$_2$R) – where we would simply find a piece of equipment that would do the job, and then stick the tubing together with sleek leukoplast waterproof adhesive tape, no pressure alarms, no alarms associated with the system at all.[191] The accepted view would be: 'Well, it's okay, because the patient's going to die anyway if we don't do it.' I think that has changed considerably. I don't know if people would agree with me over that, but I think that's been a real major move.

Bion: Not only risk, but also a gradual, somewhat reluctant, acceptance of the fact that standardization of the best practice is better than Brownian motion. But it's a very slow process.

Wright: On a personal note: I came back from Australia, having had six months there and been exposed to critical incident reporting in anaesthesia. When I returned in 1988, we opened a new ICU in the Western General Hospital in Edinburgh and in 1991 I published a paper of our experience of critical incident reporting in intensive care.[192] So there was an awareness

---

[190] Dr David Morrison wrote: 'Safety wasn't a terribly important consideration in the early days. It must be remembered that we had taken on the business of rescuing the dying, that there were no real rules in the pioneering days, and that the public respected what we were attempting to do and were not so litigious. As experimental techniques became routine treatment and as rules became defined, criteria of safety were developed. Bio-engineering research highlighted some of the problems of electrical safety and Hospital Technical Memorandum no. 8 (HTM8), the technicians' bible, was one of the early standards documents. See Department of Health and Social Security (1963).' From 'Development of ICUs', document written in response to a letter from a nursing officer doing a research project in ICU history, 1992. Original document will be deposited along with other records of the meeting in archives and manuscripts, Wellcome Library, London, in GC/253. HTM8 was superseded by the British Standard BS 5724 part 1, in 1979. For further background on electrical safety, see McCarthy *et al.* (1974).

[191] For a review of these treatments, see, for example, Lewandowski (2000); Lanigan and Withington (1991).

[192] Wright *et al.* (1991).

of it, but it took another decade before people grasped that. If I could raise another point, which is about Joe's mention of a document relating, or detailing the structure of an ICU.[193] There were documents relating to the physical construction of ICUs and we certainly used those in the setting up of the ICU in the Western. I'm not sure if anybody here was involved in those, these were standards for light and services and bed space, and things like that? Was anybody here involved in the construction of the drawing up of those early documents?[194]

Adam: Very early on when I was a senior nurse in the Middlesex ICU, I was approached by the Department of Health nursing officer, whose name I forget now, and asked to comment on the proposals that were being put together for those health building notes. I think it was HBN27.[195] They were very, very detailed, weren't they? Absolutely. But a good first step.

Haynes: The World Health Organization did produce a quite substantive document relating to the design of intensive care units in the late 1960s.[196]

Ashworth: May I make a comment about the Department of Health guidelines for intensive care? When we first built the unit in Liverpool, one of the things everybody commented on was the space we had, because knowing that we needed space, we had 200 square feet per bed, plus circulating space. And everybody said, 'But you can't have that much!' We said, 'That's okay, the Department of Health's not paying for it.' It was a Nuffield-funded unit. But a year or two later, it was in the DHSS guidelines that this was the space required, and it was important.[197]

Another interesting thing that happened: a little later than that, was that the Department of Health decided on having what they called a 'harness unit

---

[193] See page 44.

[194] Ms Pat Ashworth wrote: 'We justified it on the basis of effective working, reduced cross-infection risk and less stressful environment. The Broadgreen ITU was designed with cushioned flooring and acoustic ceiling tiles, and pale blue and grey curtains, floor etc., to encourage a peaceful atmosphere, given the known problems of some ITUs.' Note on draft transcript, 7 September 2010.

[195] See Intensive Care Society (1997).

[196] Working Group on Intensive Care for Respiratory Insufficiency (1977).

[197] Hospital Building Note 27 (HBN27) was first published by the DHSS in 1967, updated in 1970 and 1974. The most recent edition, as Health Building Note 27, was published in 1992 and is the main planning guide used in the UK.

hospital' and this was a design of a hospital and its individual units.[198] The idea was that somebody could take either the whole hospital or individual units, and because Liverpool was thought to have some expertise in intensive care, we were asked to do the bit of the intensive care unit.

Hutton: There are two groups we haven't talked about in the development of intensive care in the UK: technicians and physiotherapists. And I don't think we actually have any here today, which is a pity, but I wonder if we could get a few views? My impression of physiotherapists was that they were much more important in the past than they seem to be at the moment, but that may be wrong.

Bion: They are more important but they're only just beginning to understand why.

Singer: Absolutely. I think they have completely re-badged their role. Somebody made a comment earlier about thumping chests now being a thing of the past. Physiotherapists have now realized that they offer very little benefit by doing that. Their major role at present is in rehabilitating and mobilizing the patient. We're now sometimes good at saving life, though sometimes we simply prolong death. Many of these patients are incredibly wasted, as a function of their critical illness, so the ability to be mobile and fit enough to cope on a general ward is now a fundamental core role of the physio. This is very different to what it was ten years ago.[199]

Hutton: What about in the development of intensive care units? Do people feel physios are important? In general, lots of nodding.

Browne: The physiotherapists were very important members of the intensive care unit team as, apart from other things, they dealt with the management of bronchial secretions. When I first went to Massachusetts General, Henning Pontoppidan had just appointed his first physiotherapist, who had been trained in the UK, and everyone on the unit was very impressed with the results of her treatment of the patients on the unit; it revolutionized the management of patients.

Strunin: I agree that they were the people who taught everybody else in the unit how to do proper suction and all the rest of it. In order to get it right,

---

[198] For a discussion of hospital planning, see Francis *et al.* (1999), in particular page 34 about the harness system.

[199] See Appendix 4, pages 105–06.

though, I got the workshop to make a plastic model of the head of the hospital's administration, and we made it into a model so that you could do suction on it. [Laughter] It was extremely lifelike and we published it in the *British Medical Journal* and people used to write to ask for copies of the paper, so if you look through the *BMJ,* you'll see a plastic model of the then head – no names – of the management of the hospital.[200]

Haynes: The first physiotherapist who was specifically unit-orientated was at the Middlesex, as far as I was concerned, and her name was Sue Lewis. She worked as part of the multidisciplinary team and actually helped set up, if not establish, a physiotherapy course for intensive care patients, or rather, for physiotherapists. Prior to that I'd always been used to weaning patients off ventilation and it was always, as far as I was concerned, a nursing responsibility. But, forgive me, part of the multidisciplinary team. [Laughter] A lot of the physical weaning of patients became a physiotherapy responsibility.[201]

Wright: Another key role for physiotherapists, particularly those who had worked in ICU, was the ability to spot patients who should be receiving attention from intensive care staff in the wards, and in what became high-dependency areas.

Sykes: To go back to the technicians. In the early days, I think that a lot of the ventilators were very poorly constructed and we relied very heavily on a man in our instrument workshop to look after them. At the Hammersmith Hospital we initially had very few ventilators. We then discovered that there were two Engström ventilators in Birmingham that had been purchased by the Ministry of Health to treat polio in the mid-1950s but that no one knew how to use them, so we went up there in a van and brought them back to Hammersmith. The instrument technician and I then spent several weeks rebuilding them and working out how they worked and they continued to serve us well for many years. The other problem was the sterilization of the ventilators. We went through a period in the 1960s when many patients became infected and

---

[200] Hilliar and Strunin (1974).

[201] Ms Pat Ashworth wrote: 'It was a number of years before we had any physiotherapists around much "out of hours", not surprisingly as there was one very good physio for the 100+ cardiothoracic patients as well as the ITU in Broadgreen Hospital.…before we started an ICU, I, a ward sister, was already used to teaching breathing exercises to our cardiothoracic surgery ward patients before an operation when our one physio for the 100-bed unit was on holiday. I certainly had no ambitions to take on more! (Remember in those days almost all of our staff were students.) Unfortunately everyone always seems to have thought that nurses can go on indefinitely taking on the work of others, from cleaners to doctors and those in between, and it still happens, I'm sure.' Letter to Mrs Lois Reynolds, 7 September 2010; e-mail, 29 March 2011.

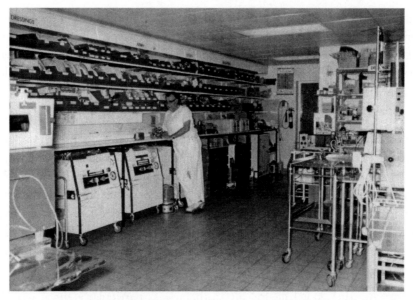

Figure 15: The technician at Royal Victoria Infirmary, Newcastle upon Tyne, showing the two dialysis machines and two Cape ventilators (foreground) for which he cared, 1982.

we started to use sterile suction catheters and 'no-touch' techniques,[202] but we were left with the problem of how to sterilize the ventilators. We started off by circulating ethylene oxide or formalin vapour, and we had to have a man to carry out this process. When we came to the use of autoclavable circuits the technicians were not so essential, but many of us kept our technicians for they had become a very valuable part of the whole set up.

Hutton: Were they officially classed as clinical workers?

Sykes: They were physics technicians, I think. They were very lowly graded and they were very badly paid.[203]

Stoddart: Yes, the trouble with the technician in an intensive care unit is that he has to be a polymath. We found a wonderful polymath in a man, who'd been injured in a mining accident (some of his fingers were missing) and he

---

[202] For a description of a 'no-touch' technique for tracheal suction, see Sykes (1960); see also note 200.

[203] Clinical scientists work either directly with patients or support clinical staff; their professional status was recognized by setting up the Clinical Scientists Board through the Professions Supplementary to Medicine Act 1960. For further details on NHS requirements, including descriptions of early qualifications, see www.rmpd.org.uk/faqs/clinical_scientists_careers.htm (visited 21 March 2011).

wanted to do something. He came into the intensive care unit and was taught on the job, to clean, service and to sterilize equipment and he became an expert at mixing the right solution for dialysis, for example. I have a photograph somewhere showing him with a bucket and a wooden stirrer turning this solution round with his hand.[204] I don't know whether there is a training course for intensive care technicians now, or whether each of the specialties must have its own technician. But this man did absolutely everything (Figure 15). Even better than that, he was a wonderful dancer and taught the nurses how to dance. [Laughter]

Wright: Going back a bit further, another key role for technicians was doing blood gas investigations, certainly in the Royal Infirmary, Edinburgh, in 1961 when the intensive care unit – or assisted ventilation unit – was set up. Shortly after that there was an anaesthetic technician whose prime role was doing blood gas investigations. The relationship of people like this with the clinical chemistry department was very important for maintaining standards. That sort of technician was later replaced by modern equipment, but they must have played a very key role in the 1960s, 1970s and early 1980s.

Gilbertson: Keith just said they were very poorly paid. I think perhaps in this Witness Seminar we ought to mention this because our theatre technicians, who as Keith said, sterilized our ventilators and always had one ready when we wanted it, did a myriad of things that they weren't paid for at all. They were actually theatre technicians and we, because I was in charge of the anaesthetic department as well, were able to persuade a couple of them to take interest in intensive care, and they were absolutely invaluable. They had no career prospects, no career structure, but they did it out of the goodness of their hearts. Another hopelessly underpaid person who was critical to our intensive care unit, or critical care unit, I suppose, was Mary, who was a nursing assistant. She undertook to do all the ordering of supplies for us. We had sort of a pool of so many drip sets and so many Swan–Ganz catheters and so many CVP lines, and when it got down to a critical level, Mary would order some more. She was paid as a nursing assistant. So I think a lot of us relied on good will from these people and we had no reason to suspect that they would or to expect that they would do it.

Singer: There are two further groups I'd like to throw into the equation: dieticians and pharmacists, who are integrated very much into the multidisciplinary team

---

[204] For a further example of making solutions for dialysis, see Crowther *et al.* (eds.) (2009): 43.

and basically check that we are doing the right thing. For example, there is now such a plethora of drugs and interactions: renal failure, liver failure, etc.[205] The UK is very well developed compared to mainland Europe. For example, there's even a UK Critical Care Pharmacists' Association.[206]

Browne: I wish to reinforce the comments people have made about technicians. Dominic Cox, who originally came to the Royal Free as an operating department technician, then came to work with us on the newly developing three to six-bedded ITU in 1974/5.[207] He was responsible for the management of ventilator equipment, blood gas and electrolyte analysis machines, the introduction of the thrombo-elastograph (TEG) monitoring equipment, the collection of data for scoring systems and data analysis, computer records and research projects. His contribution to the Royal Free intensive care unit was outstanding.

Ashworth: I would like to support the importance of the dieticians, even in the early days, having worked in an intensive care unit where there was no dietician in the hospital. The medics knew that they wanted low-salt diets for some of the cardiac patients, but if you asked them how many grams they wanted, they hadn't a clue. So, periodically, I used to spend a good portion my life working out what to do for the necessary diets.

Wright: I'm not sure whether this was just an Edinburgh phenomenon, but we always had a bacteriologist, who had a close relationship with the unit. From 1961 there was a bacteriologist associated with the unit in the Royal Infirmary, and we had one in the Western as well. It was a key role.

Ledingham: The same was true in our unit with radiology. Interpretation of all the various X-rays that were taken in the ITU required specialized knowledge of the care that these patients were receiving. In the end, we had a specific radiologist who was responsible exclusively for the interpretation of the ITU X-rays.

---

[205] See Reynolds and Tansey (eds) (2008a): 62; (2008b): 34, 63–9.

[206] For international comparisons, see Dager *et al.* (2010). The United Kingdom Clinical Pharmacy Association, established in 1981 with the aim of supporting and encouraging the emergence of clinical pharmacy, also has a critical care group, see www.ukcpa.org/ (visited 12 April 2011).

[207] Dr Doreen Browne wrote: 'When I took up my consultant post at the Royal Free in 1971, the enlightened head of the physiotherapy department, Miss van Leuthin, allotted a full-time physiotherapist to the unit whose role in those days was focussed on respiratory management. Dominic Cox's role developed along the lines of the respiratory technicians who I had seen at Massachusetts General. He went on to qualify as a clinical scientist.' Note on draft transcript, 11 September 2010.

Hutton: Perhaps if we could switch a little bit now to ethics on the intensive care unit. Margaret, you were kindly going to say a few words about this.

Branthwaite: If we look back at the beginning of intensive care, in, say, the 1950s, it is probably fair to say that none of us were taught anything about ethics then, and medicine was a paternalistic subject: doctor knows best. Since that time, medicine has become infinitely more complex and has the capacity to create harm as well as benefit. At the same time, patients have become more sophisticated and want to have their say in what is done. Julian has already referred to the fact that there is a conflict over resources, and these problems are common to medicine as a whole. But intensive care, perhaps, has brought more focus on some of the ethical disciplines, for two reasons. First of all, it is often previously healthy adults who become acutely sick. Such patients were legally incompetent. But perhaps the most important of all is the proximity, in time, between the decision taken and the outcome. If chemotherapy is withdrawn from somebody with leukaemia, the outcome may not be entirely clear – how the death is going to occur nor when. If you discontinue mechanical ventilation in somebody who can't breathe, the outcome is very immediate and there in front of you. So intensive care, to some extent, became a focal point for the emergence of ethics as a conflict in medicine.

One of the good things about this was that it made teams more multidisciplinary. I happen to have come from a unit where there were plenty of prima donnas, very cardiac surgical, it wasn't at all multidisciplinary until that was fought for and only after I had virtually left did it reach that stage. But nevertheless, even somewhere like the Brompton, pressure from patients or families meant that treatment recommendations were not exclusively medical; it was a team effort. That was one step forward.

But ultimately some of these issues were so contentious, particularly those relating to paediatrics, that it was necessary to go outside the realms of the clinical decision-makers. Partly that was done through ethics committees within hospitals. Even then, there was still conflict, so it was inevitable that the matter went to the lawyers. You may say: 'Well, what on earth did they know about medicine?' The answer is: nothing. Nevertheless, society empowers the law-makers with the responsibility for resolving disputes between parties. That, I suggest, is how the law became involved in the resolution of disputes that had arisen as ethical conflicts within a medical setting.

Initially the lawyers loved this and they grabbed it to themselves and were prepared to offer ethical advice and discuss the morals of it all. 'Yes', they said, 'it was difficult' and they felt it was a very weighty and onerous responsibility, but nevertheless they did it. Gradually, it became more and more a feature – particularly of the 1990s – that difficult cases were referred to the courts, who would then decide, and that was alright, wasn't it? Eventually even the lawyers thought: 'Well, actually, we are no better equipped to resolve ethical dilemmas than you doctors. We haven't got any special ethical training. We are not endowed with some extra power for differentiating right from wrong.' So there was a peak, as it were, of the willingness of the law to say: 'You'll do this; and you'll do that; and you'll not do the other.' There has been a pulling back in the recent past, manifest perhaps most accurately in a single case concerning the withdrawal of treatment from an extensively paralysed child about 18 months old. An application was made by the hospital for the termination of mechanical ventilation and it was opposed by the parents.It was the judge who said: 'If, as a matter of law, I find it is in the best interest of this child that treatment should be withdrawn, it is then lawful for you to do so. The fact that I tell you that it's lawful doesn't mean that you have to do it. The ethical decision, Doctor, rests with you.'[208]

My point is that medical ethics started off as a result of pressure from families and, to some extent, from patients. It became contentious, it went to the lawyers and some very useful guidelines have emerged, which I, for one, feel grateful, even if it is only in retrospect. But the lawyers have also recognized that they too have no overwhelming power to resolve these dilemmas. They will give you guidelines; the concept of 'best interests' goes far beyond the purely medical. They will say: 'What we believe, as a matter of law, is in the best interests of this patient, having listened to the evidence from all sorts of people, but the application of the ethical principles goes back to you.' I am comfortable with that, and I hope that most of you are too.

I was also asked to comment on 'outreach', high dependency and follow-up – all of them rather different. As far as outreach goes, in a way Ron Bradley and his trolley trundling around the wards was a form of outreach. [Laughter] The way the term is used now, of course, is that it can prevent too much pressure on the valuable intensive care beds – it is a question of expertise from the intensive care unit going out to see patients on the general wards, to advise on how treatment might be better implemented, or maybe to try to prevent somebody who's a bit borderline from deteriorating to the point where they need to come into the

---

[208] For details of the case An NHS Trust v MB [2006] EWHC 507 (Fam), see www.familylawweek.co.uk/ site.aspx?i=ed2067 (visited 21 March 2011); see also, for example, Powell (2007).

ICU. This approach has been greatly helped by the fact that other disciplines do now recognize that intensive care does actually have something to offer.

As far as high dependency goes – it says here 1990 to 2000 (Table 1) – I think high dependency goes back far, far longer than that. The Brompton's medical high dependency unit (HDU), the Blunt ward, opened, I think, in about 1972 or 1973.[209] HDUs started as multicentre facilities, governed by the sort of 'need' that existed in that particular hospital. Ours was a need for severe acute asthma, because these patients almost always have their crises in the early hours of the morning when wards are least well-staffed; these patients are scattered all over the place, you had to run from here to there and if you usually get there too late, they were likely to be brain damaged, because they're already anoxic when they arrest.[210] We gathered all these patients together in an HDU. The crucial thing about high-dependency, to my mind, is that it does not require one-to-one nursing care, and whether you put it a step down from the postoperative recovery room or a step down from ICU, the concept is still the same. I think somebody used the term 'stage-two beds', but it is a step down from the most intensive facility.[211]

In terms of follow-up, I would pay tribute here to the nurses, because, to me, they were the people who first recognized that perhaps families and patients had lived through a quite punishing experience and maybe it didn't all end when they left the doors of the intensive care unit, or even the doors of the hospital. One of the things, even in my day, and goodness knows I left it 20 years ago, was the realization that patients and their relatives saw the intensive care experience quite differently from how we had believed that to be. Sometimes they thought it was far worse; sometimes they actually thought it wasn't half as bad and they were terribly grateful, so that if anybody had said: 'Oh, that's awful, we don't want to go on with that,' they would have said: 'No, not so at all.' A final tribute would be to the people at the department of primary health care, University of Oxford, who have produced the follow-up site for DIPEx, a survey of the reactions of patients and their relatives to an intensive care experience, where you can log in to this site and watch video recordings of interviews with people

---

[209] Hetzel *et al.* (1977).

[210] Cochrane and Clark (1975). For an analysis of asthma admissions to the Brompton Hospital (January 1974– June 1976), see Hetzel *et al.* (1977).

[211] For the classification of individual patient dependency introduced in 2000 by the Department of Health, see Appendix 4, page 106.

who were willing to share their experiences.[212] Here is a resource for those who are suddenly forced into intensive care through some accident or ill health and feel completely overwhelmed and want a bit of assistance. This is something that I think all doctors ought to support, but which has come from disciplines other than medicine.

Adam: I think outreach is an area that grew principally from the comprehensive critical care review. It was recognized just prior to that in 1998, the Audit Commission Report showed that patients weren't being recognized early, or being followed up for that matter.[213] They are two sides of the same coin, if you like. Wards were not always in the best place to recognize patients that needed either admission or readmission to intensive care. There was a proliferation of outreach as a result of that particular report. The other point is that I can remember when Mervyn Singer and I were doing our paper about why patients died on wards, there were numerous events that could clearly have been prevented.[214] There were avoidable deaths around. That is why outreach was grasped so singularly and put in place so prolifically across the nation.

Branthwaite: I think one of the things that has made outreach so popular is that, with the changes in the working timetable of junior staff, the continuity on the general wards for all disciplines is now so much less, whereas at least with the throughput of staff on the intensive care unit, you can take that expertise into almost any area of the hospital at any time.

Ashworth: Could I go back to ethics for a moment? As soon as cardiopulmonary resuscitation with external massage became possible, that presented a problem for nurses, which was when to resuscitate and when not? Unfortunately it didn't get any better when we started with intensive care units. It was: when to resuscitate and when not to? Many medical staff had a great resistance to the idea of ever writing 'not for resuscitation'. Some patients could be resuscitated and with some it was obviously never going to be successful. But it was the nurse usually who was present when it happened. She was in great danger of being criticized if she did resuscitate, because after all the patient was going

---

[212] The Database of Individual Personal Experiences (DIPEx) is a charity founded by Drs Ann McPherson and Andrew Herxheimer in 2001 and works closely with the Health Experiences Research Group, University of Oxford. In 2008, the DIPEx website was relaunched as www.healthtalkonline.org, covering people's experiences of over 60 health conditions (visited 15 April 2011).

[213] Audit Commission (1999); Dawson and McEwen (2005).

[214] McGloin *et al.* (1999).

to die; or being criticized because she hadn't, because the patient had arrested and she should have done resuscitation. I remember, because we had had some experience by this time with the two-bed intensive care unit. I was asked to go down to North Wales to talk about this around 1962–64. I realized that I had opened my mouth to talk about it because many of the doctors and nurses talking about these patients didn't understand what was going on, unless you had actually had these patients – before the definition of brain death.[215] And these patients were not such as most of us had seen before. I found that in North Wales I was faced not only with nurses but the local Roman Catholic priest and a young doctor who said, 'But that it made him feel like a murderer if he was asked to write "not for resuscitation".' I said at that time, 'Well, you know, as a surgeon, that people say: "this patient is not suitable for operation; they're inoperable" – why is it different?' The consequence, as was said earlier, was that the result happens much quicker.[216] But I truly hope by now that the nurses don't have the same problem in critical care units and that there is clear definition as to who is and who is not to be resuscitated.

Ledingham: Sticking with ethics, Peter – I'll go back a bit to the late 1960s–early1970s. The concern that we had at that time was relatively clear cut when it came to brain death and the associated decisions to withdraw life support, extubate, discontinue mechanical ventilation and so on. But my memory of the period from the late 1970s to the early 1980s was not so much about that type of patient; it concerned all the issues that Pat has talked about in relation to 'do not resuscitate' orders, etc. It was more the patient who had developed multiple organ failure, for example. We became convinced that it was relatively easy for us to keep such patients alive, and they survived – well, months would be an exaggeration – many weeks, when it was obvious and clearly accepted by everyone in the unit that this patient wasn't going to survive. But the ethical challenge for us at the time was that we, probably wrongly with hindsight, misinterpreted these problems as different from the brain-death situation. Eventually, I think it was with increasing experience that the senior doctor

---

[215] The Human Tissue Act 1961 made it easier to use organs from dead bodies by eliminating the time limit on subsequent movement and use. Section 1(4) required that the person removing a body part be a qualified medical practitioner and be satisfied that life is extinct, although no distinction was made between being 'legally dead' and 'medically dead'. Removal of organs required consent, given by the deceased before death or by those in possession of the body, effectively the relatives at home or the coroner in hospital with the relatives' consent. This legal concept of death was determined in 1968 as a result of the early heart transplants in Britain. See Tansey and Reynolds (1999): 32–4, 38, 39; see also Jennett (1980, 1994).

[216] For further discussion, see page 74.

and the senior nurse would take a decision that we were going to discontinue treatment at some point earlier than had happened in years gone by. Then the issue of the family consultation arose and so on. That was a major ethical issue for us in the 1970s.

Bion: I think that gradually there is a much more sophisticated understanding of the nature of risk and uncertainty in the professions and in the public, but it's a very slow process. The other change that has occurred, as Margaret has reflected on, is that care is now not so much mandated as negotiated and I think that is important. There's much more transparency now, so that the decisions 'not to resuscitate' have to be documented, and documented very clearly. And we have to be advised. I think that's an asset too. Finally, as part of that, the outreach process helps to identify patients who should not be put through the burdens of intensive care. It's one of the major benefits of having an outreach service far in advance of any other aspect of what they might deliver. We learn about that because we now follow-up our patients. We've introduced such a process in our hospital, including the family satisfaction survey.[217] We get information back from that which empowers us not to apply excessive burdens given the perception of a highly significant risk of an adverse outcome with continued care.

Ball: I want to add something to the previous speaker's point in relation to the decision-making in intensive care now. Because we have such a lack of continuity due to the European working time directive, in my experience sometimes people don't look at the one piece of the chart, or on the computer where it says 'day 160'. What they do is to look at the physiology and say: 'Oh yes, I can tweak that bit. I can treat that little bit of physiology. I can do something about the ventilator.' But they don't look at the bigger picture, because often it's easier not to, when you are there at an ITU for a day or three, and then you're gone again for quite a considerable time in some cases. So I think that is a problem that we now have, and no doubt we'll find a solution in the future.

Gilbertson: I was interested in what you were saying, and I particularly sympathized with Iain Ledingham. It is quite easy over several months to accumulate a ward full of patients who have been there for weeks with no room for more acute patients. I think the only way out of that in the 1960s, 1970s and 1980s was by the more experienced clinicians. I used to write my 'Sunday think'. I'd go in on a Sunday and look through the whole unit and see what

---

[217] See, for example, Bright *et al.* (2004); see also note 167.

was going on. It became evident that although some of the patients had had everything we had to offer, it still hadn't worked, and it was time not to offer anything else aggressive. Two senior people – myself and Peter Drury – used to make it a point that we would talk to the relatives and explain: 'Look, we've tried everything else, all the antibiotics, and now your aunt is going into renal failure and we honestly don't think we should dialyze. But we promise, you know, if she does die, we'll keep her comfortable.' I never, never had any relatives who wouldn't accept a reasonable explanation like that. As the staff of the unit grew from just me to three people, to five people, to seven people – the more junior consultants found it very difficult to accept that. It's one of the reasons I retired in the end; I rather became sickened of the futility.

To comment on Pat's Roman Catholic priest in Wales. I don't know every Roman Catholic priest in Wales, but I never found any conflict with the fact that I was a Roman Catholic and stopping treating when it was futile. I would certainly not subscribe to euthanasia, certainly not just before the Pope's visit (Pope Benedict XVI visited England and Scotland, 16–19 September 2010) [Laughter], but futile treatment is no part of any Christian discipline that I know of.

Bion: Judaism permits withholding of treatment, but not active withdrawal of life-sustaining treatment. Indeed, it is reported that mechanical ventilators in Israel now incorporate a timer, which can be set to stop ventilators automatically so that the clinicians can 'withdraw' by not having to re-start futile treatment.[218]

Hutton: Yes, well, there are a number of variants on that in different sects. I seem to remember, because I haven't done intensive care *per se* for some time now, that in the 1980s there was quite an important paper that demonstrated the longer somebody stays in intensive care, the more you spend, and the less likely there will be a successful outome.[219] And that quite a large proportion of the total intensive care bill was spent on futility.

Bion: Yes, the greatest expenditure is on the non-survivors. But long-stay: no. That is a much more complex issue, much more complex. Often we simply haven't understood the nature of what chronic critical illness is. We are beginning to understand it now, but the data is quite confusing. You don't necessarily have worse outcomes because you've been there for three months, except that,

---

[218] Ravitsky (2005).

[219] See, for example, King's Fund Panel (1989); Gilbertson *et al.* (1991).

of course, futility and the attitude of mind that you've just mentioned, is the reason that people finally give up and pull the plug, and then, of course, you have a self-fulfilling prophecy.

Adam: May I say that I'm talking about 'follow-up'. Does anyone want to continue the debate about ethics and so on?

Strunin: I am going to support Julian there. I got him to write an editorial for me for the *British Journal of Anaesthesia* – he's probably forgotten this – I couldn't believe it when I read it: 'The most expensive patients in intensive care are the ones who die.'[220] I remember reading that and asking: 'Is that actually accurate?' You convinced me that it was, and you were right. Obviously if the patient gets better and leaves, that is cheaper than if they stay.

Singer: I've been doing this job for 25 years and in that time I've witnessed a few major changes. We now have a greater ability to prolong death. To echo Julian's point, I think patients now generally die of therapeutic fatigue rather than our inability to keep them alive. So, it is more of a conscious decision to pull out or not escalate, despite the ability to do so.[221] From my experience, we are now far less paternalistic – decisions used to be made on behalf of the patient but now there is far more involvement of the patient and his/her family. I think this is absolutely right, but now, if anything, it is perhaps swinging too much the other way. I spend a large amount of time trying to manage the patients' and relatives' expectations. They see the majority surviving on television programmes such as *House* and *Holby City*.[222] Medics also talk up what is possible, especially the -ologists. The change has not been particularly subtle, but more of a quantum shift in the way we manage patients and the way we manage death. There was a wonderful paper from Iain Ledingham in the *Lancet* on septic shock.[223] Iain looked at how patients died in Glasgow over a three-year period; and showed that the average time to death shifted from very early to day 5–7. Please correct me if I'm wrong, Iain, but your article was written as a triumph, an achievement, that we were keeping the patients alive to die later on. Nowadays the 100-day patient stay isn't that unusual. It is certainly a different environment from that I experienced when I started practising intensive care.

---

[220] Bion and Strunin (1996); Bion (1995).

[221] See, for example, British Medical Association (1999); Thomas (2003).

[222] See, for example, Casarett *et al.* (2005); see also Braakman *et al.* (1988).

[223] Ledingham (1978).

Adam: Moving on from that slightly, we are aware that about 20 per cent of our patients, having been in intensive care, die having been transferred out to the ward, if that makes sense? things to which I would like to pay tribute is that this follow-up process that has actually reduced the mortality rate of these patients, or we think it has. On top of that, I'd like to pay tribute to Richard Griffiths and Christina Jones who have put so much work into understanding the impact of critical care on patients and their families, and have put so much effort into ameliorating the problems overall.[224] That work has been going for at least ten years, maybe 15 years, I would say, and thus has contributed, I hope, to improved outcomes.

Wright: I'd be interested in people's observations on mortality over this 25–30-year period looking backwards, in that it hasn't changed as dramatically as one would have hoped, and that's because with the expansion of intensive care units and the increasing expectations, we've gone for sicker and sicker patients. That's a surprising thing that the mortality hasn't improved as much as you would have hoped in that time.

Bion: There is a black box. The black box is chronic disease and lack of physiological reserve. That is almost an immeasurable and presents us with real difficulties. When you measure acute illness, severity of disease, APACHE scoring,[225] it's this composite between the magnitude of the insult and the sophistication of the support. And, you don't know what the reserve is. Very often that comes through when taking a clinical history and observing the patient's passage over time. That's one of the things that I think has changed. We are taking more patients with less reserve, whether you measure that as advanced age or co-morbid disease. There are many different ways of doing it, but we don't have a very good way of measuring it.

Singer: To echo that point, when I was a medical registrar the local cardiac centre would not take a patient for coronary artery bypass surgery if they were aged 60 years and one day, I remember doctoring the notes to make the patient younger. [Laughter] Now age is no bar and certainly in the 11 years of ICNARC's existence, the mean patient age has gone up by one year, every year.

Strunin: When Hillary Clinton, First Lady of the US, attempted to revise US healthcare in 1994, she went round intensive care units in the US and went to

---

[224] See, for example, Griffiths and Jones (2007).

[225] Knaus *et al.* (1985, 1991).

an enormous unit where you couldn't see the patients for equipment. She asked: 'Why are these patients here?' They replied: 'Well, these are very sick patients and we're going to make them better.' She then said: 'Will they all get better?' The intensivist said: 'I'm afraid they won't.' She replied: 'How much will it cost to make them better?' And he said: 'It's not a matter of money – they have things we can't deal with.' The next question, which he couldn't answer – nor was there an answer: 'Why are they here?'

Ledingham: For the record, this is in response to David's earlier query.[226] Just before I left this country for a sojourn in the Middle East in 1988, I was one of a group of people invited by the King's Fund to discuss and comment on outcomes from intensive care. The people who were there included Bryan Jennett and Joe Stoddart, with Professor John Ledingham from Oxford in the chair.

If my memory serves me correctly it was surprisingly difficult for the group to produce evidence that intensive care had lowered mortality in any of the groups of conditions that the panel had been invited to consider.[227] I take Julian's point that things have moved on since then, but it was a disquieting experience for those of us round the table, most of whom had been in the business for 20 or 30 years. To be aware that scientific evidence suggested that our endeavours were not actually saving lives was, not surprisingly, a source of concern.

Hutton: Do you think there's a sort of moving average among the profession that allows people into intensive care, which produces a relatively stable mortality rate? Do you understand what I mean? I don't do intensive care any more, but I do preoperative assessment clinics in high-risk patients, many of whom don't even start the path to surgery because we've turned them away. I think part of you needs to say: 'Well, what's the chance of this?' Obviously it would be wasteful to take everybody, but you have to draw a line somewhere. I have to say that where I draw the line depends, obviously, on the individual – it is a personal decision between you and them – but I think we have a moving average of what is possible with technology and medicine that will produce a mortality rate that we would feel is worth aiming for. I suspect that, in some ways, that the mean value has been maintained, but the quality of the patients coming in has become more complex.

---

[226] See page 81.

[227] King's Fund Panel (1989).

Ledingham: I agree and, to quote a specific example of acute concern to me towards the end of the 1980s, there was an awareness that certain surgical conditions were almost inevitably going to lead to death. I'm thinking, for example, about ruptured abdominal aortic aneurysm in the elderly patient. I come from a surgical background so it was relatively easy for me to discuss these issues with surgeons. Nevertheless, there was a great reluctance on the part of my surgical colleagues not to operate on such patients after they had discussed the prognosis with the family. Yes, they could carry out a procedure that could be acutely life saving: 'It would be a matter thereafter for the intensive care people to make sure the patient left the hospital alive', which we knew from our records that we were extremely unlikely to be able to do.

Bion: This leads us to the general question: do intensivists do any good? And of course there's a large body of data which says, 'Yes', as you would expect, because that's what we want to see. There is one single, very large US study published by Mitchell Levy, based on observational database of over 100 000 patients where the answer is 'No'.[228] I think the truth lies between the two; I'm confident that we do do good, but it's very difficult to measure. We have huge capacity to do harm and we have to factor that into all our conversations with families, because it's much, much easier to make things worse than to make them better.

Spencer: I'm going to have to leave the meeting shortly, because I have a longish way to go, but I did want to add a little anecdote to all this conversation about standardization in intensive care units. In about 1982 I crossed the Atlantic to New York to see a neurologist who was working in a hospital in the middle of the East River, the Goldwater Memorial Hospital, which was called by the Americans a 'chronic facility'. She had developed a method of giving nocturnal respiratory aid to paralysed people using a nosepiece. We had tried that and failed. Within five minutes it was quite clear what she was doing that we were not, and we very quickly learnt how to do it as a result of that trip. She knew that in the remote past I had had a mild reputation in intensive care and I was invited to go and see their intensive care unit. I was very reluctant because I wanted to get back home, but one has to be courteous, so I went. This was a unit of 42 beds. Every single patient in the unit was naked and aged over 80; they all had tracheostomies, and were being ventilated by positive pressure. I said, 'Well, as I get older, one of the things that I find myself doing in London is giving advice to people running intensive care units on how to prevent this sort of thing from happening.' 'Oh', she said, 'you mustn't do that.' And I thought:

---

[228] See Levy *et al.* (2008); see also Vincent *et al.* (2010).

'My goodness me, this woman has some strange religious beliefs', which, I believe, do exist in America. She said: 'No, no. We're a chronic facility. We accept ventilator-dependent patients from all hospitals and intensive care units within New York. And because we can make economies of scale, if we keep these people alive, we can make a profit on doing so, which funds the unit which you've crossed the Atlantic to see.'

Singer: A very quick follow-up on Julian's point about the harm we inflict on our patients. A major change in the last 10–15 years in intensive care has been the introduction of large, multicentre, academic trials that are not industry-driven. Time and again they've shown that many of the therapies we provide to the patient causes harm.[229] Thus, the major advances in intensive care in the last ten years have been, to my mind, partly process – we're far better at process – but also in doing less. We ventilate less hard, we sedate less hard, we give less blood, we're trying to give fewer drugs to keep the blood pressure at physiologically meaningless figures. We're now appreciating the concept of doing less harm to the patient. Simply because we've got the ability to make the numbers look normal, does not confer benefit. The physiology of a chronic critically ill patient is very different to that of a healthy person.

Gilbertson: To go back slightly, not to whether we do good or harm, but to whether we can tell which it is that we're going to do. When I was five years from retirement, I divided my contract into two halves and I kept half as a clinical anaesthetist and in the other half I had time to do research, looking at what we'd done in the previous 20 years. We kept very careful notes; we had APACHE scores and every other sort of score on every patient for a very long time. I learnt – in fact I paid £40 to a statistician to help me with all this, my own money – to produce these receiver operating characteristic curves, which balance sensitivity against specificity of various admission characteristics of our patients.[230] There were 30 or 40 of them; it varied from time to time. It was very disappointing, because we could never find any characteristic or group of characteristics because we did univariate and multivariate analysis. We could never find any characteristic or group of characteristics that would tell us whether the patient was going to die in intensive care. We could get within 10

---

[229] For examples of conventional practice being harmful, see Hébert *et al.* (1999); Brower *et al.* (2004); Girard *et al.* (2008).

[230] From signal detection theory, these curves were used to make sense of noise-contaminated radio signals and have become attractive in medical decision-making. For a review of decision-making tools, see Fischer *et al.* (2003).

per cent, 7 per cent, maybe 5 per cent, but all my colleagues said: 'Well, are you going to refuse a person a 5 per cent chance of saving their life by not admitting them?' The answer is 'no'. Statistics don't work like that. They don't work for individuals. It would be marvellous if we could confidently predict whether or not we could save a particular patient, not least because it has been shown that patients who die cost more than patients who survive.[231] But we could never forecast who we should not admit.

Hutton: Okay, I think that's a suitable point, perhaps, to draw this to a close. Thanks to everybody and Tilli has a few comments to make.

Tansey: Like Peter, I would like to say thank you very much to you all for coming. It's been a fascinating afternoon. I think we've actually raised more questions than we've answered, and there may be a possibility of holding an additional Witness Seminar with some of these other voices we're missing today: the physiotherapists, the technicians and the patients. And this may be a job for another organization like the Intensive Care Society, or one of the Royal Colleges, because one of the things that comes from these meetings are spin-off meetings. I'd particularly like to thank my team: Wendy Kutner, who has been in touch with you all in setting up this meeting; and Lois Reynolds and Ania Crowther, who have been carrying the microphones around. I'd particularly like to thank Peter Hutton for chairing this meeting. Perhaps you hadn't realized that he was on take last night and this morning when a new hospital opened in Birmingham and he was on call at 2am this morning. So we're very grateful to you, Peter, for coming down and chairing this Witness Seminar. And perhaps you'll all join us for a glass of wine.

---

[231] See, for example, Detsky *et al.* (1981).

Appendix 1

Dr Alan Gilston's draft structure for the Intensive Care Society, 1970[237]

Suggested title: "The Intensive Care Society"

Need for its creation

There are a large number of active specialist societies, witness the number of surgical clubs and societies. In anaesthesia too there are already several specialist societies apart from the College of Surgeons and the Association.

Intensive Care Units now play an essential role in the care of the gravely ill. They are also becoming more numerous. At the moment the exchange of information between different centres and different disciplines is at best haphazard and it depends on the occasional article (often in a specialist journal), symposium, lecture or personal contact. Improvement in the exchange of information must surely benefit the patient since few physicians are completely familiar with the management of every grave derangement of the vital organs.

Present Societies clearly cannot satisfy this need.

Aims and functions of the Society

1.   The collection and dissemination of information on Intensive Care. This includes techniques, research in progress or results, reviews of the literature, and recent advances in management and equipment.

2.   Discussion of problems, whether clinical, research, organisational or political.

---

[237] Stoddart (2005); reproduced by permission of the Intensive Care Society.

3.   Establishment of combined projects.

4.   Evaluation of new apparatus.

5.   To provide expert advice for new Units and for various interested organisations, manufacturers or persons, both here and abroad.

6.   To form specialist subcommittees to explore specific problems and advise the Society.

Membership

1.   All members must be of Consultant rank, or its equivalent, and intimately engaged in Intensive Care work.

2.   Membership must be open to all disciplines and this must be actively encouraged for it is fundamental to the aims of the Society.

3.   The initial membership should be limited to say forty, (?) with a maximum of eighty (?) members, not more than five new members being elected in one year. There is a danger of unlimited membership preventing the personal informal contact which is essential for the Society's success. It would also present problems in administration and might not allow the invitation of guests.

4.   If there are over forty (?) applications for immediate membership, election should be made by the founding ad hoc committee and based on the candidates standing and on the natu of his publications and work. Thereafter membership should be by election at the AGM of the Society on the basis of these criteria.

5. A maximum of two members per Unit.

6. The success and viability of the Society will demand that its members be actively engaged in Intensive Care work. To make room for younger colleagues members must retire on reaching the age of 55.

7. Honorary life membership may be bestowed on distinguished candidates, who need not necessarily be members of the Society.

8. Suitable provision should be made for the exceptional need to suspend a Member from the Society. Failure to pay the subscription is the most likely problem.

Committee

1. This should consist of say seven persons, namely:

    Chairman
    Secretary
    Treasurer
    Research Officer
    Three co-opted members

2. Initially it should be an ad hoc committee for administrative convenience and for the selection of members if immediate applications exceed forty (?).

3. Whilst it might be desirable from some points of view that a completely fresh committee should be appointed after say the first two years, this would be administratively unsatisfactory and some form of continuity should be devised either in the duration of tenure of say the office of chairman or secretary or in the "staggering" of retirements.

4.   Future elections for Office should be made at the AGM.

5.   No office should be held for a total of more than four years, to prevent "greybeard" domination of the Society.

Meetings

These should be held not more than twice per year.

2.   If possible they should be held in the provinces as well as in London. At the moment members will inevitably pay their own expenses. *Hughes*

3.   ~~Their content should be decided by the Society's~~ Committee. *1 Mill*

4.   They should aim at attracting the interest of most members.

5.   If funds permit, one or more guest speakers should be invited to address the Society. They should receive first class expenses and where possible, an honorarium.

6.   The meetings should be as informal as possible.

Finance

1.   ~~Drug and instrument firms~~ should be ~~approached for Endowment funds.~~ Should the Society become well-established ~~they~~ might also support research projects, guest speakers and other expenses.

2.   A membership/fee of two or perhaps three guineas per annum would probably cover administrative expenses. This would be allowable for Income Tax purposes after

registration of the Society.

Legal Expenses

These would arise with the registration of the Society as a Charity for Income Tax and other purposes.

Appendix 2

Outline curriculum in general intensive care nursing for State Registered Nurses, Course Number 100[237]

Aim of the course

To train registered nurses in all aspects of general intensive care nursing.

General information

Entry requirements: The course is for nurses registered on the general or sick children's Register for England and Wales, Scotland or Northern Ireland. It is recommended that each nurse should have a minimum of six months' experience (not necessarily in the specialty) as a staff nurse before taking the course.

Length of the course: The period of training shall be 24–27 weeks, exclusive of any holiday during the course.

Teaching time: Not less than the equivalent of a total of 28 days shall be devoted to the planned teaching programme (which excludes one-to-one clinical teaching) commencing with an introductory period of five days, during which time the nurses will be given details of all aspects of the course, orientated to the hospital, have preparatory induction into the work of the intensive therapy unit and gradual introduction into the unit team.

Clinical experience: Clinical experience shall be gained chiefly in :-

i. a main general intensive therapy unit of not less than 6 beds

ii. a series of specialized intensive therapy units which will provide experience in the skills outlined in the curriculum. The amount of time spent in anyone unit shall be in proportion to the depth of knowledge and level of skill required.

Clinical experience shall also include short visits to other departments relevant to the course.

Assessment of course members: There should be progressive assessment of skills, knowledge and attitudes throughout the course rather than one final

---

[237] This outline curriculum, *c.* 1974, was donated by Ms Pat Ashworth and will be deposited in archives and manuscripts, Wellcome Library, London, in GC/253 along with other records of the meeting.

examination. The most important skills will need to be tested formally and in detail at the appropriate point in the course, whereas others may be recorded after supervised practice. Knowledge should also be tested at the appropriate point in the course. Attitudes are difficult to assess, but there should be an appraisal of the behaviour towards patients, relatives and colleagues which is appropriate to the attitudes outlined in the curriculum.

Night duty: Not more than one-quarter of the total length of the course shall be spent on night duty. Health authorities will be free to make their own arrangements for the night duty undertaken by nurses during the course, but these arrangements must fit suitably into the overall educational pattern of the clinical and theoretical programme. Account should be taken of the number of permanent night staff employed in the unit and the adequacy of the supervision available at night.

Holidays: Course members will be entitled to their normal leave while undertaking this course. It is recommended that some holiday should be given about half-way through the course. Holidays should be arranged to fit suitably into the overall pattern of the clinical and theoretical programme.

Sick leave and special leave: In deciding whether or not sick leave and special leave should be made up at the end of the course, health authorities will consider each case on its own merits. Long periods of absence will generally necessitate the nurse restarting the course.

Management topics (Objective 4): Attention is drawn to HM(69)2 and the report of the National Nursing Staff Committee on management development of nurses. Staff concerned with teaching this part of the curriculum should preferably themselves have had first-line and middle-management training.

Use of a schedule: It is recommended that a schedule be prepared in which to record practical instruction, practice under supervision and progressive assessments.

Library services: A selected list of books should be prepared for the nurses' use. A wide range of reference books and journals on all related topics and some of the books listed must be readily available in the library. A list of some of the books published in the specialty is on pages 12–15 (see page 98).

Objective 1

At the end of the course the nurse will be skilled in giving total nursing care to patients undergoing intensive therapy.

Skills	Knowledge	Attitudes
	History, development and scope of intensive care.	Shows interest in and willingness to participate in all aspects of the course.
	Special aspects: psychological ethical and medico-legal.	Appreciates the importance of high standards of nursing care.
	The intensive care team and the role of the nurse.	Appreciates the teamwork necessary for successful patient care.
		Respects the human dignity of every patient and his relatives.
Special procedure for admission and transfer of patients.		Behaves maturely in situations of stress and shows awareness of the emotional stress in the intensive care situation and its effects on the patients, their relatives and the staff.
Application and adaptation of nursing skills.	Special features of nursing patients in the intensive therapy unit.	
The use of specialized equipment and its application for investigation and treatment.	The use and management of specialized equipment.	Is aware of the suffering of patients and their relatives and their need for sympathy and understanding.
	Hazards of monitoring and other equipment.	
Lifting, moving and positioning patients attached to machines, instruments or appliances.	Body mechanics.	
	Measurement techniques.	
Supplementary physiotherapy.	Active and passive movements and the complications of immobility.	
Aseptic techniques in intensive care situations.	Cross infection, its prevention and treatment.	Appreciates the importance of high standards of aseptic discipline and practice.
Monitoring of response to drug therapy.	Special drugs used in intensive therapy.	
Special nursing care and management of patients being nursed in the unit.	Applied anatomy and physiology of body systems.	
	Symptoms, investigation, assessment and management of patients	

Skills	Knowledge	Attitudes
	commonly nursed in the unit.	
*Intravenous therapy including massive blood transfusions.	**Metabolism**	
	Normal nutritional needs.	
	Normal bodyfluids: electrolyte balance, acid: base balance, fluid balance.	
	Metabolic changes and their correction.	
Venepuncture for taking specimens.	**Circulatory system**	
	Circulatory dynamics:	
*Arterial puncture.	hyper- and hypo-volaemia and their correction	
*Central venous pressure.		
Expired air resuscitation.		
External cardiac compression.	arterial and venous blood pressure hyper- and hypo-tension and their assessment and correction.	
Electrocardiography, application of electrodes and the use of oscilloscopes.		
	Cardiac arrest and its treatment.	
	Electrocardiography, dysrhythmias, their interpretation and treatment.	
Emergency defibrillation.	The use and management of defibrillators and pacemakers.	
	Principles and purpose of cardiac catheterization and pacemaking.	
	Other relevant disorders and their treatment.	
Use of artificial airways and endotracheal intubation.	**Respiratory system**	
	Relevant disorders and their treatment.	
Care of tracheostomy tubes.		
Aspiration and use of suction apparatus.	Methods and hazards of intubation.	
Use of oxygen equipment and humidification.	Tracheostomy, care and management.	

* The role of the nurse will usually be to prepare the patient and equipment, assist the doctor and give after-care.

Skills	Knowledge	Attitudes
Use of lung ventilators and breathing assistors. *Bronchoscopy.	Principles, uses and management of lung ventilators and breathing assistors. The principles and methods of chest drainage.	Is aware of the psychological and psychiatric needs of the suicidal patient and shows a sympathetic understanding of the problem.
*Chest drainage. The care and management of underwater seal drainage.	**Renal system** Relevant disorders and their treatment. Blood biochemistry relating to dialysis.	
*Peritoneal dialysis.	Principles and methods of peritoneal and haemodialysis.	
Nursing care and management of the unconscious patient.	**Nervous and endocrine systems** Relevant disorders and their treatment.	
Care and management of major trauma.	**Skeletal system and soft tissue** Relevant disorders and their treatment. Major trauma and its complications.	
Care and management of acute poisoning.	**Other emergencies** e.g. acute poisoning. **Principles of intensive care applied to children**	

* The role of the nurse will usually be to prepare the patient and equipment, assist the doctor and give after-care.

Objective 2

At the end, of the course the nurse will be skilled in making clinical observations, taking measurements, interpreting these and taking appropriate action.

Skills	Knowledge	Attitudes
Noting change in the patient's condition. Observations and measurements including: continuous assessment of the changing condition of the patient reading monitors and other instruments accurately interpreting observations and determining appropriate action recording and reporting maintenance of records.	Recognition of physical and psychological changes in the patients. Clinical and other observations and their interpretation.	Appreciates the importance of comprehensive observation in the intensive care situation.

Objective 3

At the end of the course the nurse will be skilled in communication and in establishing good relationships with the patient and his family and with colleagues.

Skills	Knowledge	Attitudes

Human relationship skills.
Effective communication with:
  patients
  relatives
  colleagues
  the unit team
  staff from other parts of the hospital.
	The psychology of human relationships.
	
	Factors which contribute to good relationships.
	
	Communication techniques.
	
	The effects of breakdown in communication.
		Appreciates the importance of establishing good relationships and communication.

Objective 4

At the end of the course the nurse will have an understanding of: the management and organization of the unit; the principles of design of an intensive therapy unit and an appreciation of research.

Skills	Knowledge	Attitudes
Planning and carrying out total care of one patient.	Organization of the unit including:	Accepts responsibility.
Planning and carrying out total care of a group of patients.	policies in the unit;	Appreciates the importance of teamwork.
Organising and supervising the work of others and giving verbal and written instructions.	organization of patient care;	
	deployment and control of staff;	
Making verbal and written reports on patients.	provision and maintenance of supplies and equipment;	
Taking charge of the unit.	maintenance of records;	Appreciates the value of research and its contribution to better patient care.
	care of property and valuables.	
	Purpose and design of the unit including services and equipment.	
Recording data and information.	Maintenance of fabric and services.	
	Introduction to the principles and methods of research.	
	Ethical implications of research and treatments including organ transplant.	
	Evaluation of new equipment and materials.	
	Development of new procedures and techniques.	

Objective 5

At the end of the course the nurse will have an understanding of basic methods of learning and teaching and will be able to pass on skills and knowledge effectively to staff.

Skills	Knowledge	Attitudes
Application of teaching methods to the teaching of students and other staff.	Methods of learning and teaching.	Appreciates the importance of teaching others and is willing to accept this responsibility.
		Accepts responsibility for continuing professional self-development.

Book list

ADAMS J C. *Outline of Orthopaedics.* Williams & Wilkins. 1967 (US).

ALSTEAD S & GIRDWOOD R H. *Textbook of Medical Treatment.* Churchill Livingstone, 1974.

ASHWORTH P M & ROSE H. *Cardiovascular Disorders.* Bailliere Tindall. 1973.

ASPINALL M J. *Nursing the Open-Heart Surgery Patient.* McGraw Hill, 1973.

BAIN W H & WATT J K. *Cardio-Vascular Surgery.* Livingstone. 1970.

BENDER M B. *Approach to Diagnosis in Modern Neurology.* Grune, 1967 (US).

BENDIXON H H. *Respiratory Care.* Kimpton, 1966.

BETSCHMAN L I. *Handbook of Recovery Room Nursing.* F D Davies, Philadelphia.

BIRCH A A. *Emergencies in Medical Practice.* Churchill Livingstone, 1971.

BOYD W. *Textbook of Pathology.* Lea & Febiger, 1970.

BRAIMBRIDGE M V. *Postoperative Cardiac Intensive Care.* Blackwell Scientific, 1974.

BURRELL Z L & BURRELL L O. *Intensive Nursing Care.* Saint Louis, Mosby, 1969.

CAMERON J S & RUSSELL A M E. *Nephrology for Nurses.* Heinemann, 1970.

CAMPBELL E J M, *et al. Clinical Physiology.* Blackwell, 1971.

CLARKE D B & BARNES A D. *Intensive Care for Nurses.* Oxford, Blackwell, 1971.

CLELAND W. *Medical & Surgical Cardiology.* Blackwell, 1969.

CONWAY N. *A Pocket Atlas of Arrhythmias.* Wolfe Medical, 1974.

CRAMER, SANNERSTEDT, THULIUS & WERKO. *Cardiac Arrhythmias and Quinidine.*

CRUIKSHANK R. *Medical Microbiology.* Williams & Wilkins, 1965 (UK).

DAVIES B D & OTHERS. *Microbiology.* Harper & Row, 1970.

EMERY E K J, YATES A K & MOORHEAD P J. *Principles of Intensive Care.* English Univ. Press, 1973.

FARMAN J V. *Anaesthesia & the EMO System.* English Univ. Press, 1973.

FELDMAN S A. *Muscle Relaxants.* W B Saunders, 1973 (US).

FELDMAN S A & ELLIS H. *Principles of Resuscitation.* Blackwell, 1967.

FELDMAN S A & CRAWLEY B E. *Tracheostomy & Artificial Ventilation in the Treatment of Respiratory Failure.* Arnold, 1971.

FINN R & DRURY P M E. *Guide to the Intensive Therapy Unit.* Butterworth, 1974.

FLEMING J S & BRAIMBRIDGE M V. *Lecture Notes on Cardiology.* Blackwell, 1974.

GARROD L P, LAMBERT H P & O'GRADY F. *Antibiotic and Chemotherapy.* Churchill Livingstone, 1973.

GERSON G. *Intensive Care.* Heinemann, 1973.

GILSTON A & RESNEKOV L. *Cardio-Respiratory Resuscitation.* Heinemann Medical, 1971.

GOODMAN S &GILMAN A. *The Pharmacological Basis of Therapeutics.* Collier Macmillan, 1970.

GREEN PROF. J H. *Introduction to Human Physiology.* Oxford Press, 1972.

HAMPTON J R. *The ECG Made Easy.* Churchill Livingstone, 1973.

HARVARD C W H. *Current Medical Treatment.* Staples Press, 1970.

HARVEY J R. *The Kidney & the Internal Environment.* Chapman & Hall, 1974.

HERSHEY S G & OTHERS. *Septic Shock in Man.* Little, 1971 (US).

HITCHCOCK E R & MASSON A H B. *Management of the Unconscious Patient.* Blackwell, 1970.

HOPKIN D A B. *Anaesthesia. Recovery & Intensive Care.* English Univ. Press, 1970.

HUBNER P J B. *Nurses' Guide to Cardiac Monitoring.* Bailliere Tindall, 1971.

HUNTER A R. *Essentials of Artificial Ventilation of the Lungs.* Churchill, 1966.

JENNETI N B. *An Introduction to Neurosurgery.* Heinemann, 1970.

JONES R S & OWEN-THOMAS J B. *Care of the Critically Ill Child.* Arnold, 1971.

JULIAN D H. *Cardiology.* Bailliere Tindall, 1970.

KELMAN, G. R., *Physiology: A Clinical Approach.* Churchill Livingstone, 1972.

KELMAN G R. *Applied Cardio-Vascular Physiology.* Butterworth, 1971.

LAING J G & HARVEY J. *The Management & Nursing of Burns.* English Univ. Press, 1971.

LASCELLES P T & DONALDSON D. *Essential Diagnostic Tests.* Medical Technical Press, 1970.

LONDON P S. *Practical Guide to the Care of the Injured.* Livingstone, 1967.

MATHEW H & LAWSON A A H. *Treatment of Common Acute Poisonings.* Churchill, 1971.

McNAUGHT A B & CALLENDER R. *Illustrated Physiology.* Livingstone, 1970.

MELTZER L E *et al. Concepts and Practice of Intensive Care for Nurse Specialists.* Charles Press. 1969.

MELTZER L E *et al. Intensive Coronary Care: A Manual for Nurses.* Charles Press, 1965.

METHENY S M & SNIVELY W D. *Nurses' Handbook of Fluid Balance.* Lippincot, 1967.

MOLLINSON P L. *Blood Transfusions.* Blackwell, 1972.

MOUNTJOY P & WYTHE B. *Nursing Care of the Unconscious Patient.* Bailliere Tindall, 1970.

MUSHIN W W *et al. Automatic Ventilation of the Lung.* Blackwell Scientific, 1969.

NOBLE, CHAMBERLAIN, COULSHED & RUBIN. *Elementary Cardiography.*

NORRIS W & CAMPBELL D. *Anaesthetics, resuscitation and intensive care: A textbook for students and residents.* Edinburgh, Livingstone, 1971.

NORRIS W & CAMPBELL O. *A Nurses' Guide to Anaesthetics, Resuscitation & Intensive Care.* Livingstone, 1969.

NOTTER L E. *Essentials of Nursing Research.* Springer, New York, 1974.

NUNN J F. *Applied Respiratory Physiology.* Butterworth, 1969.

OLSZOWKA A J. *Blood Gases.* Lea & Febiger, 1973.

OSTLERE G & BRYCE-SMITH R. *Anaesthetics for Medical Students.* Churchill Livingstone, 1972.

PONTOPPIDAN, GRIFFIN & LOWENSTEIN. *Acute Respiratory Failure in the Adult.*

POTTER J M. *The Practical Management of Head Injuries.* Lloyd-Luke, 1974.

RICKHAM P P & JOHNSTON J H. *Neonatal Surgery.* Butterworths, 1969.

ROBERTS K D & EDWARDS J M. *Paediatric Intensive Care.* Blackwell, 1971.

ROLLASON W N. *Electrocardiography for the Anaesthetist.* Blackwell, 1969.

RUSSELL W J. *Central Venous Pressure.* Butterworths, 1974.

SCHAMROTH L. *Introduction to Electro-cardiography.* Blackwell, 1971.

SMITH S. *How Drugs Act.* Macmillan Journals, 1971.

SPALDING, CRAMPTON-SMITH. *Clinical Practice and Physiology of Artificial Respiration.*

STOCK J P P. *Diagnosis and Treatment of Cardiac Arrhythmias.* Butterworths, 1970.

STORLIE F. *et al. Principles of Intensive Nursing Care.* Appleton-Century Crofts, New York, 1970.

SYKES M K, McNICHOLL M W & CAMPBELL E J M. *Respiratory Failure.* Blackwell, 1969.

TAYLOR W H. *Fluid Therapy.* Blackwell, 1970.

THACKER E W. *Postural Drainage and Respiratory Control.* Lloyd-Luke, 1971.

TURNER R W D. *Electrocardiography.* Livingstone, 1964.

ULDHALL R. *Renal Nursing.* Blackwell Scientific, 1972.

WADDINGTON P J. *Physiotherapy in Artificial Respiration.* Livingstone, 1969.

WAHLIN A, WESTERMARK L & VAN DER VLET A. *Intensive Care.* Wiley, 1974.

WALTER W F & JOHNSTON I D A. *Metabolic Basis of Surgical Care.* Heinemann Medical, 1971.

WEST J B. *Respiratory Physiology.* Blackwell Scientific, 1974.

WHELPTON D. *Renal Dialysis.* Sceptre Pubs., 1974.

WILKINSON A W. *Parenteral Nutrition.*

WILKINSON A W. *Body Fluids in Surgery.* Livingstone, 1969.

WILSON F. *Tracheostomy for the Nurse.* Arnold, 1970.

WOOD P. *Diseases of the Heart & Circulation.* Eyre & Spottiswood, 1968.

WOOD-SMITH, VICKERS & STEWART. *Drugs in Anaesthetic Practice.* Butterworths, 1968.

WORLD HEALTH ORGANISATION, REGIONAL OFFICE FOR EUROPE. *Nursing In Intensive Care.* Report on a Seminar covered by Regional Officer for Europe. Copenhagen, WHO, 1971.

Appendix 3

Excerpt from 'Priorities in the use of physiotherapy' by the Chartered Society of Physiotherapy, c. 1970[237]

PRIORITIES IN THE USE OF PHYSIOTHERAPY

Note by the Chartered Society of Physiotherapy for
discussion with representatives of certain branches
of the Medical Profession.

1.   For many years the number of physiotherapists in the National Health
Service, expressed as whole-time equivalents, has increased very slowly,
whilst the demand for their services has been rising at a much higher rate.
The current demand cannot be fully met and the Society wishes to discuss,
informally in the first instance, with representatives of those branches of
the medical profession most concerned the possibility of establishing priorities
in the use of physiotherapy.

2.   Discussion could range over a wide field and in order to try to reach
useful conclusions it is proposed to confine attention, at present, to the
following topics:-

3.   Intensive Care

    3.1.   The establishment of an increasing number of intensive care
    units has led to the demand that physiotherapists should be available
    to assist in the postural drainage and aspiration of bronchial
    secretions at frequent intervals throughout the day and night.

    3.2.   At the same time there has been an increasing demand for
    physiotherapists to fill a similar role in the management of acute
    respiratory lesions in medical wards and after certain surgical
    operations.

    3.3.   Unlike nurses who cover 24 hours in shifts physiotherapists are
    organised to cover the day shift only but within their physical
    capacity, they have willingly done overtime to treat urgent cases.
    However, if physiotherapists work an evening or night shift they have
    to be given time off duty the following day and, because of the
    shortage of physiotherapists, this results in about 20 in-patients or
    out-patients being deprived of treatment. Moreover, an increasing
    and now substantial proportion of the physiotherapy staff of hospitals
    are married women, many of whom cannot undertake night duty or even
    work full time all day because of their family commitments so that the
    burden of night duty has to be carried by unmarried staff. This
    burden has become so great that it must be eased.

---

[237]   Ms Pat Ashworth wrote: 'I would guess I acquired the document above around the late 1960s–
early 1970s, as it was with my papers of the Royal College of Nursing intensive therapy nursing group.
One does wonder whether they thought all night nurses were unmarried and without children or
other family responsibilities, which they certainly were not in our ITU.' Letter to Mrs Lois Reynolds,
7 September 2010.

3.4.   <u>Questions</u>(a) Is the expertise of the physiotherapist essential or at least highly desirable, in intensive care? Or (b) should nurses be trained to take over full responsibility for this work? Or (c) should nurses and physiotherapists be trained to do this work, the latter being responsible for training the former and helping them in the management of especially difficult cases?

3.5.   If (c) is the best practical compromise is it reasonable to limit the responsibility of physiotherapists, save for very exceptional cases, to the period from 8 a.m. to 11 p.m. so that they cover the change-over of the day and night nursing staff?

3.6.   It will be impossible to provide sufficient physiotherapists to cover (c) unless economies in the use of their time in other directions can be effected.

Appendix 4

Intensive care and high dependency: definitions

Guidelines on admission to and discharge from intensive care and high dependency units, Department of Health, March 1996[237]

Intensive care is appropriate for:	High dependency care is appropriate for:
Patients requiring or likely to require advanced respiratory support alone (e.g. IPPV)	Patients requiring support for a single failing organ system, but excluding those needing advanced respiratory support
Patients requiring support of two or more organ systems	Patients who can benefit from more detailed observation or monitoring than can safely be provided on a general ward
Patients with chronic impairment of one or more systems sufficient to restrict daily activities (co-morbidity) and who require support for an acute reversible failure of another organ system	Patients no longer needing intensive care, but who are not yet well enough to be returned to a general ward Postoperative patients who need close observation or monitoring for longer than a few hours

---

[237] Department of Health: *Comprehensive Critical Care* (2000).

Classification of individual patient dependency introduced in 2000, Department of Health[238]

Level 0	Patients whose needs can be met through normal ward care in an acute hospital
Level 1	Patients at risk of their condition deteriorating or those recently relocated from higher levels of care, whose needs can be met on an acute ward with additional advice and support from the critical care team
Level 2	Patients requiring more detailed observation or intervention, including support for a single failing organ system or postoperative care, and those stepping down from higher levels of care
Level 3	Patients requiring advanced respiratory support alone or basic respiratory support, together with the support of at least two organ systems. This level to include all complex patients requiring support for multiorgan failure

---

[238]   From page 2 www.ics.ac.uk/intensive_care_professional/standards_and_guidelines/standards_for_intensive_care_2007 (visited 18 February 2011).

Appendix 5

Twenty-four *Nursing Times* articles claiming a nursing contribution to the establishment of intensive care units, arranged by date, 1965–98

collated by Dr Tony Gilbertson[237]

Author	Date	Title	*Nursing Times* reference
Fisher B	**1965**	A patient with cerebral hypoxia nursed in an intensive care unit	**61**: 1470–2
Anon.	**1965a**	Tutors and intensive care	**61**: 1564
Anon.	**1965b**	Intensive care units	**61**: 1804–5
Anon.	**1965c**	An intensive therapy chart	**61**: 1650–1
Davies D	**1966**	Infective polyneuritis. 1. In the intensive care unit	**62**: 141–3
Pearce D J	**1966**	Intensive care unit of Southampton General Hospital	**62**: 146
Anon.	**1966a**	Intensive care	**62**: 674–5
Anon.	**1966b**	Intensive care and internal communications	**62**: 659
Hothersall T	**1966**	Intensive care unit; a nurse administrator's view	**62**: 760–3
Anon.	**1966c**	The hospital centre: nurse planning meetings; intensive care units	**62**: 887–8
Anon.	**1966d**	Acute care ward; Charing Cross Hospital, London	**62**: 1126–7
High M	**1967**	Chest and liver: multiple injuries: a case history illustrating intensive therapy	**63**: 1580–3

[237] For discussion, see page 22.

Author	Date	Title	*Nursing Times* reference
Irvine M	**1968**	Progressive patient care in Northern Ireland	**64**: 185–6
Parker D J	**1969**	Intensive therapy after cardiac surgery	**65**: 341–2
Davies M	**1969**	Chickenpox complicated by pneumonia. A problem in intensive care	**65**: 487–90
McCartney A	**1969**	A nursing care study: myocardial infarction	**65**: 1549–50
Morley A, Spark M	**1970**	The nurse and machine-dependent patient	**66**: 849–52
Dobson M	**1970**	The coronary care unit: patients' attitudes and the role of the nurse	**66**: 869–71
Quarrell E J	**1970**	Artificial ventilation. 3. Nursing care	**66**: 1360–2
Postle M	**1971**	Faecal peritonitis complicated by severe chest infection – a patient care study	**67**: 630–3
Lennon M	**1971**	Coronary care in Belfast	**67**: 921–4
McAlister E	**1972**	A respiratory and intensive care unit	**68**: 203–4
Finn B	**1973**	Post-basic training in renal nursing	**69**: 833
Payne D	**1998**	Awesome foursome	**94**: 12–13

References

AA, GH, JY. (1985) Obituary: H R Youngman. *British Medical Journal* **290**: 326.

Adam S K, Osborne S. (1997) *Critical Care Nursing: Science and practice.* Oxford: Oxford University Press.

Adams E B, Holloway R, Thambiran A K, Desai S D. (1966) Usefulness of intermittent positive-pressure respiration in the treatment of tetanus. *Lancet* **ii**: 1176–80.

Adams E B, Wright R, Berman E, Laurence D R. (1959) Treatment of tetanus with chlorpromazine and barbiturates. *Lancet* **i**: 755–7.

Amin D K, Shah P K, Swan H J C. (1986a) The Swan–Ganz catheter: choosing and using the equipment. *Journal of Critical Illness* **1**: 34–7.

Amin D K, Shah P K, Swan H J C. (1986b) The Swan–Ganz catheter: insertion technique. *Journal of Critical Illness* **1**: 38–45.

Amin D K, Shah P K, Swan H J C. (1986c) The Swan–Ganz catheter: tips on interpreting results. *Journal of Critical Illness* **1**: 40–8.

Amin D K, Shah P K, Swan H J C. (1986d) The Swan–Ganz catheter: indications for insertion. *Journal of Critical Illness* **1**: 54–61.

Angus D C. (2008) Introduction: Scoring systems. In Fink M, Hayes M, Soni N. (eds) *Classic Papers in Critical Care*, 2nd edn. London: Springer-Verlag: 449.

Anon. (1961) Editorial: the Platt report. *British Medical Journal* (15 July): 159.

Anon. (1965a) Editorial: tutors and intensive care. *Nursing Times* **61**: 1564.

Anon. (1965b) Editorial: Intensive care units. *Nursing Times* **61**: 1804–5.

Anon. (1965c) Editorial: An intensive therapy chart. *Nursing Times* **61**: 1650–1.

Anon. (1966a) Intensive care. *Nursing Times* **62**: 674–5.

Anon. (1966b) Intensive care and internal communications. *Nursing Times* **62**: 659.

Anon. (1966c) The hospital centre: nurse planning meetings; intensive care units. *Nursing Times* **62**: 887–8.

Anon. (1966d) Acute care ward; Charing Cross Hospital, London. *Nursing Times* **62**: 1126–7.

Anon. (1983) Notes and News: Etomidate. *Lancet* **322**: 60.

Anon. (1993) Tribute to Ole Siggaard-Andersen, 60 years, 10 December 1992. *Scandinavian Journal of Clinical and Laboratory Investigation* 214 (Suppl.): 1–137.

Anon. (2010) Obituary: Alex Crampton Smith. *The Times* (7 May).

Ashbaugh D G, Bigelow D B, Petty T L, Levine B E. (1967) Acute respiratory distress in adults. *Lancet* **ii**: 319–23.

Ashworth P M. (1964) Intensive care ward: Broadgreen Hospital, Liverpool. *Nursing Times* (3 July): 867–9.

Ashworth P M. (1966) Intermittent use of the Bird respirator after cardiopulmonary bypass. *Nursing Times* **62**: 245–6.

Ashworth P M. (1976) 'Investigation into problems of communication between nurses and patients in intensive therapy/care units'. Master's thesis. Manchester: University of Manchester.

Ashworth P M. (1980) *Care to Communicate: An investigation into problems of communication between patients and nurses in intensive therapy units*, Royal College of Nursing research series. London: Royal College of Nursing.

Ashworth P M. (1990) *Bridges of Opportunity: Research linking nursing practice, education and management*, Winifred Raphael memorial lecture no. 9. London: Royal College of Nursing.

Ashworth P M, Clarke C. (eds) (1992) *Cardiovascular Intensive Care Nursing*. Edinburgh: Churchill Livingstone.

Ashworth P M, Rose H. (1973) *Cardiovascular Disorders: Patient care*, foreword by F Ronald Edwards. London: Baillière Tindall.

Ashworth P M, Richardson J C, Meadows G. (1973) Intensive therapy 1960–73: the development of a unit. *Nursing Times* (6 September): 1164–6.

Ashworth P M, Bjørn A, Déchanoz G, Delmotte N, Farmer E, Kordas A B, Kristiansen E, Kyriakidou H, Slajmer-Japelj M, Sorvettula M, Stankova M. (1987) *People's Needs for Nursing Care: A European study: a study of nursing care needs and of the planning, implementation and evaluation of care provided by nurses in two selected groups of people in the European region.* Copenhagen: World Health Organization, Regional Office for Europe. Freely available at: http://whqlibdoc.who.int/hq/1987/928901041X_(part1).pdf (visited 8 March 2011).

Atkinson B L. (1987) The intensive care unit. *Nursing* **3**: 547–51.

Atkinson B L. (1990) Training nurses for intensive care. *Intensive Care Nursing* **6**: 172–8.

Atkinson R S, Boulton T B. (eds) (1989) *The History of Anaesthesia.* International Congress and Symposium Series 134. London: Parthenon for the Royal Society of Medicine Services.

Audit Commission. (1999) *Critical to Success: The place of efficient and effective critical care services within the acute hospital.* London: Audit Commission for Local Authorities and the National Health Service in England and Wales. Freely available at www.audit-commission.gov.uk/nationalstudies/health/other/Pages/criticaltosuccess.aspx (visited 30 November 2010).

Bargh W, Griffiths H W, Slawson K B. (1967) Crush injuries of the chest. *British Medical Journal* **ii**: 131–4.

Baydur A, Layne E, Aral H, Krishnareddy N, Topacio R, Frederick G, Bodden W. (2000) Long-term non-invasive ventilation in the community for patients with musculoskeletal disorders: 46 year experience and review. *Thorax* **55**: 4–11.

Beinart J. (1987) *The History of the Nuffield Department of Anaesthetics, 1937–87.* Oxford: Oxford University Press.

Bell J A, Bradley R D, Jenkins B S, Spencer G T. (1974) Six years of multidisciplinary intensive care. *British Medical Journal* **ii**: 483–8.

Bion J. (1995) Rationing intensive care. *British Medical Journal* **310**: 682–3.

Bion J, Strunin L. (1996) Editorial: multiple organ failure: from basic science to prevention. *British Journal of Anaesthesia* **77**: 1–2.

Bion J F, Edlin S A, Ramsay G, McCabe S, Ledingham I McA. (1985) Validation of a prognostic score in critically ill patients undergoing transport. *British Medical Journal* **291**: 432–4.

Bjorneboe M, Ibsen B, Astrup P, Everberg G, Harvald B, Sottrup T, Thaysen E H, Thorshauge C. (1955) Active ventilation in the treatment of respiratory acidosis in chronic diseases of the lungs. *Lancet* **269**: 901–3.

Blagg C R. (1967) The management of acute reversible intrinsic renal failure. *Postgraduate Medical Journal* **43**: 290–306.

Boulton T B. (1989) *The Association of Anaesthetists of Great Britain and Ireland and the Development of the Specialty of Anaesthesia, 1932–92.* London: Association of Anaesthetists of Great Britain and Ireland.

Boulton T B. (2007) A career carried on the winds of medical progress. In Caton D, McGoldrick K E. (eds) *Careers in Anesthesiology: Autobiographical and posthumous memoirs, Vol. X.* Park Ridge, IL: The Wood Library-Museum of Anesthesiology: 191–300.

Boulton T B, Wilkinson D J. (1995) The origins of modern anaesthesia. In Healy T E J, Cohen P J. (eds) *Wylie and Churchill-Davidson's A Practice of Anaesthesia*, 6th edn. London: Edward Arnold: 3–35.

Bower A G, Bennett V R, Dillon J B, Axelrod B. (1950a) Investigation on the care and treatment of poliomyelitis patients. *Annals of Western Medicine and Surgery* **4**: 561–82.

Bower A G, Bennett V R, Dillon J B, Axelrod B. (1950b) Investigation on the care and treatment of poliomyelitis patients. Part 2. Physiological studies of various treatment procedures and mechanical equipment. *Annals of Western Medicine and Surgery* **4**: 687–71.

Braakman R, Jennett W B, Minderhoud J M. (1988) Prognosis of the posttraumatic vegetative state. *Acta Neurochirurgica* **95**: 49–52.

Bradley R D. (1964) Diagnostic right-heart catheterisation with miniature catheters in severely ill patients. *Lancet* **ii**: 941–2.

Bradley R D. (1977) *Studies in Acute Heart Failure.* London: Edward Arnold Ltd.

Bradley R D, Jenkins B S, Branthwaite M A. (1970) The influence of atrial pressure on cardiac performance following myocardial infarction complicated by shock. *Circulation* **42**: 827–37.

Bradley R D, Jenkins B S, Branthwaite M A. (1971) Myocardial function in acute glomerulonephritis. *Cardiovascular Research* **5**: 223–5.

Bradley R D, Spencer G T, Semple S J. (1964) Tracheostomy and artificial ventilation in the treatment of acute exacerbations of chronic lung disease. A study in 29 patients. *Lancet* **i**: 854–9.

Braimbridge M V. (1965) *Postoperative Cardiac Intensive Care.* Oxford: Blackwell Scientific Publications.

Braimbridge M V, with the collaboration of M A Branthwaite. (1972) *Postoperative Cardiac Intensive Care,* 2nd edn. Oxford: Blackwell Scientific Publications.

Branthwaite M A. (2000) *Law for Doctors: Principles and practicalities.* London: Royal Society of Medicine.

Branthwaite M A, Bradley R D. (1968) Measurement of cardiac output by thermal dilution in man. *Journal of Applied Physiology* **24**: 434–8.

Bright D, Walker W, Bion J. (2004) Clinical review: outreach – a strategy for improving the care of the acutely ill hospitalized patient. *Critical Care* **8**: 33–40.

British Medical Association. (1999) *Withholding and Withdrawing Life-prolonging Treatment. Guidance for decision-making.* London: British Medical Association.

British Medical Association, Planning Unit. (1967) *Intensive Care, planning unit report no. 1.* London: BMA.

Brodie B C. (1812) Further experiments and observations on the actions of poisons on the animal systems. *Philosophical Transactions of the Royal Society of London* **102**: 205–9.

Brower R G, Lanken P N, MacIntyre N, Matthay M A, Morris A, Ancukiewicz M, Schoenfeld D, Thompson B T; National Heart, Lung, and Blood Institute ARDS Clinical Trials Network. (2004) Higher versus lower positive end-expiratory pressures in patients with the acute respiratory distress syndrome. *New England Journal of Medicine* **351**: 327–36.

Browne D R, Davies A F, McKenzie J, Klose S. (1974) The Royal Free Hospital. 2. A mobile intensive care service. *Nursing Times* **70**: 1580–2.

Bulander R E Jr. (2010) 'The most important problem in the hospital': nursing in the development of the intensive care unit, 1950–1965. *Social History of Medicine* **23**: 621–38.

Burnett R W. (1993) Activities of the Committee on pH, Blood Gases and Electrolytes, International Federation of Clinical Chemistry, 1977–92. *Scandinavian Journal of Clinical and Laboratory Investigation* **214** (Suppl.): 41–5.

Casarett D, Fishman J M, MacMoran H J, Pickard A, Asch D A. (2005) Epidemiology and prognosis of coma in daytime television dramas. *British Medical Journal* **331**: 1537–9.

Christie D A, Tansey E M. (eds) (2004) *Cystic fibrosis.* Wellcome Witnesses to Twentieth Century Medicine, vol. 20. London: The Wellcome Trust Centre for the History of Medicine at UCL. Freely available online at www.history. qmul.ac.uk/research/modbiomed/wellcome_witnesses/

Chun G M, Ellestad M H. (1971) Perforation of the pulmonary artery by a Swan–Ganz catheter. *New England Journal of Medicine* **284**: 1041–2.

Clement A J, Hübsch S K. (1968) Chest physiotherapy by the 'bag squeezing' method: a guide to technique. *Physiotherapy* **54**: 355–9.

Cochrane G M, Clark T J H. (1975) A survey of asthma mortality in patients between ages 35 and 64 in the Greater London hospitals in 1971. *Thorax* **30**: 300–5.

Cole L B. (1934) Tetanus treated with curare. *Lancet* **ii**: 475–7.

Cole L B. (1936) The treatment of tetanus. *British Medical Journal* **i**: 1191–5.

Cole L B. (1938) The treatment and prognosis of tetanus: (section of surgery). *Proceedings of the Royal Society of Medicine* **31**: 1205–7.

Cole L B, Youngman H R. (1969) Treatment of tetanus. *Lancet* **i**: 1017–19.

Cole L B, Youngman H R, Gandy A P. (1968) An attack of tetanus. *Lancet* **ii**: 567–8.

Collier J. (2003) Obituary: Tony Dornhorst. *Guardian* (26 March).

Collier L H. (ed.) (1995) *The History of the Medical Research Club, 1891–1991.* London: Wellcome Trust for the Medical Research Club.

Committee of Nursing. (1972) *Report.* London: HMSO.

Conacher I D. (2010) The big ideas of Edgar Alexander Pask (1912–66). *Journal of Medical Biography* **18**: 44–8.

Coppel D L, Balmer H G, Dundee J W. (1973) Civil disturbance and anaesthetic workload in the Royal Victoria Hospital, Belfast. II. The respiratory and intensive care unit. *Anesthesia and Analgesia* **52**: 147–55.

Crocker C. (2007) The development of critical care in England. *Intensive and Critical Care Nursing* **23**: 323–30.

Crowther S M, Reynolds L A, Tansey E M. (eds) (2009) *History of Dialysis in the UK: c.1950–2000.* Wellcome Witnesses to Twentieth Century Medicine, vol. 37. London: The Wellcome Trust Centre for the History of Medicine at UCL. Freely available online at www.history.qmul.ac.uk/research/modbiomed/wellcome_witnesses/.

Cuthbertson B H, Sprung C L, Annane D, Chevret S, Garfield M, Goodman S, Laterre P F, Vincent J L, Freivogel K, Reinhart K, Singer M, Payen D, Weiss Y G. (2009) The effects of etomidate on adrenal responsiveness and mortality in patients with septic shock. *Intensive Care Medicine* **35**: 1868–76.

Dager W E, Shulman R, Jacobi J. (2010) Preparation and training of critical care pharmacists. In Flaatten H, Moreno R P, Putensen C, Rhodes A. (eds) *Organisation and Management of Intensive Care.* Berlin: MVV Medizinisch Wissenschaftliche Verlagsgesellschaft: 133–42.

Davies D. (1966) Infective polyneuritis. 1. In the intensive care unit. *Nursing Times* **62**: 141–3.

Davies M. (1969) Chickenpox complicated by pneumonia. A problem in intensive care. *Nursing Times* **65**: 487–90.

Dawson D, McEwen A. (2005) Critical care without walls: The role of the nurse consultant in critical care. *Intensive Critical Care Nursing* **21**: 334–43.

Department of Health, National service framework expert group. (2000) *Comprehensive Critical Care: A review of adult critical care services.* London: Department of Health.

Department of Health and Social Security. (1963) *Safety Code for Electro-medical Apparatus*, Hospital Technical Memorandum no. 8 (HTM 8). London: HMSO.

Detsky A S, Stricker S C, Mulley A G, Thibault G E. (1981) Prognosis, survival, and the expenditure of hospital resources for patients in an intensive-care unit. *New England Journal of Medicine* **305**: 667–72.

Dewar H A. (1978) The hospital nurse after Salmon and Briggs. *Journal of the Royal Society of Medicine* **71**: 399–405.

Dobson M. (1970) The coronary care unit: patients' attitudes and the role of the nurse. *Nursing Times* **66**: 869–71.

Dopson L. (2008) Peggy Nuttall: *Nursing Times'* editor unafraid to take on the medical establishment. *Independent* (21 October).

Dudley H A F. (1976) Surgical research in the UK: past, present and future. *British Journal of Surgery* **63**: 337–40.

Edwards F R, Richardson J C, Ashworth P M. (1965) Experience with an intensive-care ward. *Lancet* **i**: 855–7.

Ferris B G Jr, Pollard D S. (1960) Effect of deep and quiet breathing on pulmonary compliance in man. *Journal of Clinical Investigation* **39**: 143–9.

Finn B. (1973) Post-basic training in renal nursing. *Nursing Times* **69**: 833.

Fisher B. (1965) A patient with cerebral hypoxia nursed in an intensive care unit. *Nursing Times* **61**: 1470–2.

Fischer J E, Bachmann L M, Jaeschke R. (2003) A readers' guide to the interpretation of diagnostic test properties: clinical example of sepsis. *Intensive Care Medicine* **29**: 1043–51.

Fleming J S, Braimbridge M V. (1974) *Lecture Notes on Cardiology*, 2nd edn. Oxford: Blackwell Scientific Publications.

Florey H W, Harding H E, Fildes P. (1934) The treatment of tetanus. *Lancet* **224**: 1036–41.

Fowler K T, Hugh-Jones P. (1957) Mass spectrometry applied to clinical practice and research. *British Medical Journal* **i**: 1205–11.

Francis S, Glanville R, Noble A, Scher P. (1999) *50 Years of Ideas in Health Care Buildings*. London: Nuffield Trust.

Fraser R, Watt I, Gray C E, Ledingham I McA, Lever A F. (1984) The effect of etomidate on adrenocortical function in dogs before and during hemorrhagic shock. *Endocrinology* **115**: 2266–70.

Fricker J. (2010) Obituary: Jack Tinker. *British Medical Journal* **340**: 1247.

Ganz W, Donoso R, Marcus H S, Forrester J S, Swan H J C. (1971) A new technique for measurement of cardiac output by thermodilution in man. *American Journal of Cardiology* **27**: 392–6.

Garcias V A, Mallouh C, Park T, Stahl W M, Nagamatsu G R, Addonizio J C. (1981) Depressed myocardial function after transurethral resection of prostate. *Urology* **17**: 420–7.

Gardener M G. (1977) The history, philosophy and evaluation of the work of the Joint Board of Clinical Nursing Studies. *Journal of Advanced Nursing* **2**: 621–32.

Gilbertson A A. (1974) Pulmonary artery catheterization and wedge pressure measurement in the general intensive therapy unit. *British Journal of Anaesthesia* **46**: 97–104.

Gilbertson A A. (1995) Before intensive therapy? *Journal of the Royal Society of Medicine* **88**: 459P–63P.

Gilbertson A A, Smith J M, Mostafa S M. (1991) The cost of an intensive care unit: a prospective study. *Intensive Care Medicine* **17**: 204–8.

Gilson J C, Hugh-Jones P. (1949) The measurement of the total lung volume and breathing capacity. *Clinical Science* **7**: 185–216.

Gilston A. (1975) Report on the first world congress on intensive care, London, 24–27 June 1974. *Intensive Care Medicine* **1**: 93–7.

Gilston A. (1981) Intensive care in England and Wales: a survey of current practice, training and attitudes. *Anaesthesia* **36**: 188–93.

Girard T D, Kress J P, Fuchs B D, Thomason J W, Schweickert W D, Pun B T, Taichman D B, Dunn J G, Pohlman A S, Kinniry P A, Jackson J C, Canonico A E, Light R W, Shintani A K, Thompson J L, Gordon S M, Hall J B, Dittus R S, Bernard G R, Ely E W. (2008) Efficacy and safety of a paired sedation and ventilator weaning protocol for mechanically ventilated patients in intensive care (Awakening and Breathing Controlled trial): a randomised controlled trial. *Lancet* **371**: 126–34.

Goodman I. (1998) *The Administration of Cytotoxic Chemotherapy: Recommendations* produced by the Royal College of Nursing, in collaboration with an expert group. London: Royal College of Nursing.

Gordon I J, Jones E S. (1998a) The evolution and nursing history of a general intensive care unit (1962–83). *Intensive Critical Care Nursing* **14**: 252–7.

Gordon I J, Jones E S. (1998b) Effective clinical policies in a district general hospital. *Health Care Analysis* **6**: 295–304.

Gordon I J, van Noordwijk J, Jones E S. (2000) The first successful haemodialysis. *Journal of the Royal Society of Medicine* **93**: 266–8.

Gray R C, Coppel D L. (1975) Surgery of violence. III. Intensive care of patients with bomb blast and gunshot injuries. *British Medical Journal* **i**: 502–4.

Gray T C, Halton J. (1946) A milestone in anaesthesia?: (d-tubocurarine chloride). *Proceedings of the Royal Society of Medicine* **39**: 400–10.

Griffiths H W. (1960) Crush injuries of the chest. *Journal of the Royal College of Surgeons of Edinburgh* **6**: 13–27.

Griffiths R D, Jones C. (2007) Seven lessons from 20 years of follow-up of intensive care unit survivors. *Current Opinion in Critical Care* **13**: 508–13.

Gunning K, Rowan K. (1999) ABC of intensive care: outcome data and scoring systems. *British Medical Journal* **319**: 241–4.

Haldeman J C. (1959) *Elements of Progressive Patient Care.* Washington, DC: US Public Health Service.

Harries J R, Lawes W E. (1955) Intermittent positive-pressure respiration in bulbo-spinal poliomyelitis; use of the Radcliffe respiration pump. *British Medical Journal* **i**: 448–54.

Hartley R, O'Flynn W R, Rake M, Wooster M. (1968) Experiment in progressive patient care. *British Medical Journal* **ii**: 794–5.

Harvey S, Harrison DA, Singer M, Ashcroft J, Jones CM, Elbourne D, Brampton W, Williams D, Young D, Rowan K; PAC-Man study collaboration. (2005) Assessment of the clinical effectiveness of pulmonary artery catheters in management of patients in intensive care (PAC-Man): a randomised controlled trial. *Lancet* **366**: 472–7.

Haynes G. (1983) Nursing intensive care group journal. 2. Stress in intensive care. *Nursing Mirror* **157**: S11–12.

Hayes M A, Timmins A C, Yau E H S, Palazzo M, Hinds C J, Watson D. (1994) Elevation of systemic oxygen delivery in the treatment of critically ill patients. *New England Journal of Medicine* **330**: 1717–22.

Healthcare Industrial Liaison Group. (1987) *Directory of Emergency and Special Care Units, 1987*. St Ives, Cambs: CMA Medical Data Ltd.

Hébert P C, Wells G, Blajchman M A, Marshall J, Martin C, Pagliarello G, Tweeddale M, Schweitzer I, Yetisir E. (1999) A multicenter, randomized, controlled clinical trial of transfusion requirements in critical care. Transfusion Requirements in Critical Care Investigators, Canadian Critical Care Trials Group. *New England Journal of Medicine* **340**: 409–17. Erratum in *New England Journal of Medicine* (1999) **340**: 1056.

Hetzel M R, Clark T J H, Branthwaite M A. (1977) Asthma: analysis of sudden deaths and ventilatory arrests in hospital. *British Medical Journal* **i**: 808–11.

High M. (1967) Chest and liver: multiple injuries: a case history illustrating intensive therapy. *Nursing Times* **63**: 1580–3.

Hilliar K M, Strunin L. (1974) Teaching model for tracheal suction. *British Medical Journal* **ii**: 45.

Hoge W. (1999) Christina Foyle, 88, the queen of the London bookstore, dies. *New York Times* (June 11). See http://query.nytimes.com/gst/fullpage.html ?res=9803EED81638F932A25755C0A96F958260&sec=&spon=&pagewa nted=print (visited 8 February 2011).

Honey G E, Dwyer B E, Smith A C, Spalding J M K. (1954) Tetanus treated with tubocurarine and intermittent positive-pressure respiration. *British Medical Journal* **ii**: 442–3.

Horstmann D M. (1985) The poliomyelitis story: a scientific hegira. *Yale Journal of Biology and Medicine* **58**: 79–90.

Horton J M. (1992) A Cambridge physician and curare for tetanus. *Proceedings of the History of Anaesthesia Society* **11**: 16–21.

Hothersall T. (1966) Intensive care unit; a nurse administrator's view. *Nursing Times* **62**: 760–3.

Hugh-Jones P, West J B. (1960) Detection of bronchial and arterial obstruction by continuous gas analysis from individual lobes and segments of the lung. *Thorax* **15**: 154–64.

Hutchings A, Durand M A, Grieve R, Harrison D, Rowan K, Green J, Cairns J, Black N. (2009) Evaluation of modernisation of adult critical care services in England: time series and cost effectiveness analysis. *British Medical Journal* **339**: b4353; doi: 10.1136/bmj.b4353.

Ibsen B. (1966) Intensive therapy: background and development. *International Anesthesiology Clinics* **37**: 1–14.

Illingworth C F W, Smith G, Lawson D D, Ledingham I McA, Sharp G R, Griffiths J C, Henderson C I. (1961) Surgical and physiological observations in an experimental pressure chamber. *British Journal of Surgery* **49**: 222–7.

Intensive Care Society. (1981) *Intensive Care Yearbook 1981*. London: MMI Medical Market Information Ltd for ICS.

Intensive Care Society. (1997) *Standards for Intensive Care Units*. London: ICS. Freely available at: www.ics.ac.uk/intensive_care_professional/ standards_and_guidelines/standards_for_intensive_care_2007 (visited 18 February 2011).

Intensive Care Society. (2003) *Evolution of Intensive Care in the UK*, prepared by Saxon Ridley, Mark Dixon and members of the Intensive Care Society's Standards Committee. London: Intensive Care Society, freely available at www.ics.ac.uk/intensive_care_professional/standards_and_guidelines/ evolution_of_intensive_care_2003 (visited 31 August 2010).

Inter-Faculty Collegiate Liaison Group on Intensive Therapy. (1985) Recommendations for the training of consultants with a special interest in intensive care. *Care of the Critically Ill* **1**: 4–5.

Inter-Faculty Collegiate Liaison Group on Intensive Therapy. (1986) *Circular Letter to Postgraduate Deans.* London: Royal College of Surgeons of England.

Irvine M. (1968) Progressive patient care in Northern Ireland. *Nursing Times* **64**: 185–6.

Isberg A. (2005) Polio in focus: a personal reminiscence: the 1952 Copenhagen epidemic. *British Polio Fellowship Bulletin* (July): 12–14.

Jackson I. (1992) Bereavement follow-up service in intensive care. *Intensive Critical Care Nursing* **8**: 163–8.

Jenkins B S, Bradley R D, Branthwaite M A. (1970) Evaluation of pulmonary arterial end-diastolic pressure as an indirect estimate of left atrial mean pressure. *Circulation* **42**: 75–8.

Jenkins B S, Branthwaite M A, Bradley R D. (1973) Cardiac function after open heart surgery. Relation between the performance of the two sides of the heart. *Cardiovascular Research* **7**: 297–305.

Jenkins W J, Stone B, Knowles G S A, Tovey G H, Sharpe R A. (1959) Experiences with a disposable plastic transfusion-giving set. *Lancet* **i**: 139–43.

Jennett W B. (1980) Letter: brain death. *Lancet* **ii**: 1306.

Jennett W B. (1994) Treatment of critical illness in the elderly. *Hastings Center Report* **24**: 21–2.

Jennett W B, Ledingham I McA, Harper A M, McDowall D G, Miller J D. (1970) The effects of hyperbaric oxygen on cerebral blood flow during carotid artery surgery. In: Wada J, Iwa T. (eds) *Proceedings of the International Congress on Hyperbaric Medicine.* Tokyo: Igaku Shoin; London: Baillière, Tindall and Cassell: 469–71.

Jensen K. (1974) The poisoning treatment centre of Copenhagen. *Resuscitation* **3**: 199–204.

Joint Board of Clinical Nursing Studies. (1972) *First Report,* version 11.1. London: Department of Health and Social Security.

Joint Board of Clinical Nursing Studies. (*c.*1974) *Outline Curriculum in General Intensive Care Nursing for State Registered Nurses, Course Number 100.* London: JBCNS.

Joint Board of Clinical Nursing Studies. (1975) *Second Report.* London: JBCNS.

Joint Faculty of Intensive Care Medicine, Australian and New Zealand College of Anaesthetists and the Royal Australasian College of Physicians. (2003) Regulation 7 (1 December). See http://ama.com.au/node/3142 (visited 4 February 2011).

Jolly C, Lee J A. (1957) Post-operative observation ward. *Anaesthesia* **12**: 49–56.

Jones C, O'Donnell C. (1994) After intensive care – what then? *Intensive Critical Care Nursing* **10**: 89–92.

King's Fund Panel. (1989) Intensive care in the UK: report from the King's Fund Panel. *Anaesthesia* **44**: 428–31.

Kitson A L. (1994) *Clinical Nursing Practice Development and Research Activity in Oxford Regions, 1993*, report no. 7. Oxford: Centre for Practice Development & Research, National Institute for Nursing.

Kitson A L, Harvey G. (1991) *Bibliography of Nursing Quality Assurance and Standards of Care 1932–87*, Royal College of Nursing standards of care project. London: Scutari Press.

Knaus W A, Draper E A, Wagner D P, Zimmerman J E. (1985) APACHE II: a severity of disease classification system. *Critical Care Medicine* **13**: 818–29.

Knaus W A, Zimmerman J E, Wagner D P, Draper E A, Lawrence D E. (1981) APACHE-acute physiology and chronic health evaluation: a physiologically based classification system. *Critical Care Medicine* **9**: 591–7.

Knaus W A, Wagner D P, Draper E A, Zimmerman J E, Bergner M, Bastos P G, Sirio C A, Murphy D J, Lotring T, Damiano A, Harrell F E Jr. (1991) The APACHE III prognostic system. Risk prediction of hospital mortality for critically ill hospitalized adults. *Chest* **100**: 1619–36.

Kristensen H S. (1996) Comment on the description of the polio epidemic in Copenhagen 1952. *Acta Anesthesiologica Scandinavica* **40**: 134–5.

Lanigan C J, Withington P S. (1991) Support when gas exchange fails – ECMO, ECCO2R and IVOX. *Clinical Intensive Care* **2**: 210–16.

Lassen H C A. (1953) A preliminary report on the 1952 epidemic of poliomyelitis in Copenhagen with special reference to the treatment of acute respiratory insufficiency. *Lancet* **i**: 37–41.

Lassen H C A. (1954) The epidemic of poliomyelitis in Copenhagen, 1952. *Proceedings of the Royal Society of Medicine* **47**: 67–71.

Lassen H C A. (1956) *Management of Life-threatening Poliomyelitis, Copenhagen, 1952–56.* London: E & S Livingstone Ltd.

Laurence D R, Berman E, Scragg J N, Adams E B. (1958) A clinical trial of chlorpromazine against barbiturates in tetanus. *Lancet* **i**: 987–91.

Ledingham I McA. (1968) Hyperbaric oxygen. In Taylor S. (ed.) *Recent Advances in Surgery.* London: J & A Churchill: 295–328.

Ledingham I McA. (1972) Oxygen availability in shock. In Ledingham I McA and McAllister T. (eds) *Conference on Shock, Proceedings of a conference held at the Royal College of Physicians and Surgeons of Glasgow, 22–23 October 1970.* London: Kimpton: 52–9.

Ledingham I McA. (1978) Prospective study of the treatment of septic shock. *Lancet* **311**: 1194–7.

Ledingham I McA. (1987) Letter: intensive care: a specialty or a branch of anaesthetics? *British Medical Journal* **294**: 1095.

Ledingham I McA, McAllister T. (eds) (1972) *Conference on Shock, Proceedings of a conference held at the Royal College of Physicians and Surgeons of Glasgow, 22–23 October 1970.* London: Kimpton.

Ledingham I McA, Watt I. (1983) Influence of sedation on mortality in critically ill multiple trauma patients. *Lancet* **i**: 1270.

Ledingham I McA, Finlay W E I, Watt I, McKee J I. (1983) Letter: etomidate and adrenocortical function. *Lancet* **321**: 1434.

Ledingham I McA, Fisher W D, McArdle C S, Maddern M. (1974) The incidence of the shock syndrome in a general hospital. *Postgraduate Medical Journal* **50**: 420–4.

Ledingham I McA, McBride T I, Jennett W B, Adams J H. (1968) Fatal brain damage associated with cardiomyopathy of pregnancy, with notes on Caesarean section in a hyperbaric chamber. *British Medical Journal* **iv**: 285–7.

Leigh J M. (1974) Pulmonary circulation and ventilation. *Postgraduate Medical Journal* **50**: 562–5.

Lennon M. (1971) Coronary care in Belfast. *Nursing Times* **67**: 921–4.

Leuwer M, Ahern R, Gilbertson T. (2008) Obituary: Professor T Cecil Gray. *Independent* (26 January).

Levy M M, Rapoport J, Lemeshow S, Chalfin D B, Phillips G, Danis M. (2008) Association between critical care physician management and patient mortality in the intensive care unit. *Annals of Internal Medicine* **148**: 801–9.

Lewandowski K. (2000) Extracorporeal membrane oxygenation for severe acute respiratory failure. *Critical Care* **4**: 156–68.

Liverpool Regional Hospital Board, East Liverpool Hospital Management Committee. (1964) *Intensive Care Ward: Broadgreen Hospital,* opened on the 7 February 1964 by the Rt Hon Lord Cohen of Birkenhead, president, General Medical Council. Liverpool: Liverpool Regional Hospital Board, T Noel Mitchell, regional architect.

Lynaugh J E, Fairman J. (1992) New nurses, new spaces: a preview of the AACN History Study. *American Journal of Critical Care* **1**: 19–24.

Maag A. (1953) Polio-Smitteproblemer [Problems with the contagiousness of polio.]. *Ugeskrift for Læger* **115**: 1212–16.

McAlister E. (1972) A respiratory and intensive care unit. *Nursing Times* **68**: 203–4.

McCartney A. (1969) A nursing care study: myocardial infarction. *Nursing Times* **65**: 1549–50.

McCarthy J P, Morris J V, Whelpton D. (1974) HTM8 equipment evaluation report and test sheet. *BioMedical Engineering* **9**: 484–5.

McClelland P, Murray A E, Williams P S, van Saene H K, Gilbertson A A, Mostafa S M, Bone J M. (1990) Reducing sepsis in severe combined acute renal and respiratory failure by selective decontamination of the digestive tract. *Critical Care Medicine* **18**: 935–9.

McGloin H, Adam S K, Singer M. (1999) Unexpected deaths and referrals to intensive care of patients on general wards. Are some cases potentially avoidable? *Journal of the Royal College of Physicians of London* **33**: 255–9.

McLachlan G. (1992) *History of Nuffield Provincial Hospitals Trust: 1940–90.* London: Nuffield Provincial Hospitals Trust.

McMichael J. (1964) Obituary: Edward Peter Sharpey-Schafer. *British Heart Journal* **26**: 430–2.

MacQueen L, Kerr A B. (1974) *The Western Infirmary, 1874–1974: A century of service to Glasgow.* Glasgow: John Horn Limited.

Macrae J, McKendrick G D, Claremont J M, Sefton E M, Walley R V. (1953) The Clevedon positive-pressure respirator. *Lancet* **265**: 971–2.

Marshall J, Spalding J M K. (1953) Humidification in positive-pressure respiration for bulbospinal paralysis. *Lancet* **ii**: 1022–4.

Martin L V, Brown D T. (1988) Twenty-five years of respiratory intensive care. *Scottish Medical Journal* **33**: 233–6.

Mason S. (1966) The scope and organisation of an intensive therapy unit in a London teaching hospital. *Acta Anaesthesiologica Scandinavica* **23** (Suppl.): 117–22.

Melnick J L. (1996) Current status of poliovirus infections. *Clinical Microbiological Reviews* **9**: 293–300.

Meltzer L E, Pinneo R, Kitchell J R. (1965) *Intensive Coronary Care: A manual for nurses.* Philadelphia, PA: CCU Fund, Presbyterian Hospital in Philadelphia.

Ministry of Health, Department of Health for Scotland, Joint Working Party. (1961) *Medical Staffing Structure in the Hospital Service,* Report of the Joint Working Party. London: HMSO.

Ministry of Health and the Public Health Laboratory Service. (1962) Progressive Patient Care: Interim report of a departmental working group. *Monthly Bulletin* **21**: 218–26.

Morgan G. (1987) Letter: intensive care: a specialty or a branch of anaesthetics? *British Medical Journal* **295**: 213.

Morley A, Spark M. (1970) The nurse and machine-dependent patient. *Nursing Times* **66**: 849–52.

Mushin W W, Rendell-Baker L, Thompson P W, Mapleson W W. (1969) *Automatic Ventilation of the Lungs,* 2nd edn. Oxford: Blackwell.

Nash G, Blennerhassett J B, Pontoppidan H. (1967) Pulmonary lesions associated with oxygen therapy and artificial ventilation. *New England Journal of Medicine* **276**: 368–74.

Ness A R, Reynolds L A, Tansey E M. (eds) (2002) *Population-based Research in South Wales: The MRC Pneumoconiosis Research Unit and the MRC Epidemiology Unit.* Wellcome Witnesses to Twentieth Century Medicine, vol. 13. London: The Wellcome Trust Centre for the History of Medicine at UCL. Freely available online at www.history.qmul.ac.uk/research/modbiomed/wellcome_witnesses/

NHS Modernisation Agency. (2002) *Critical Care Programme: Weaning and long term ventilation.* Leicester: NHS Modernisation Agency.

Nilsson E. (1951) On treatment of barbiturate poisoning; a modified clinical aspect. *Acta Medica Scandinavica* **253** (Suppl.): 1–127.

Northway W H, Rosan R C, Porter D Y. (1967) Pulmonary disease following respiratory therapy of hyaline membrane disease. *New England Journal of Medicine* **276**: 357–68.

Nunn J F. (1988) The first meeting of the Anaesthetic Research Society. *British Journal of Anaesthesia* **61**: 639–41.

O'Grady N P, Alexander M, Dellinger E P, Gerberding J L, Heard S O, Maki D G, Masur H, McCormick R D, Mermel L A, Pearson M L, Raad I I, Randolph A, Weinstein R A. (2002) Guidelines for the prevention of intravascular catheter-related infections. Centers for Disease Control and Prevention. *Morbidity and Mortality Weekly Report. Recommendations and Reports* **51**(RR-10): 1–29.

Orme L. (1985) Training nurses for critical care. *Care of the Critically Ill* **1**: 6–8.

Parker D J. (1969) Intensive therapy after cardiac surgery. *Nursing Times* **65**: 341–2.

Paul J R. (1971) *A History of Poliomyelitis.* New Haven, CN; London: Yale University Press.

Payne D. (1998) Awesome foursome. *Nursing Times* **94**: 12–13.

Payne J P. (1988) Editorial I: thirty years on: anniversary of the founding of the Anaesthetic Research Society. *British Journal of Anaesthesia* **61**: 523–4.

Pearce D J. (1966) Intensive care unit of Southampton General Hospital. *Nursing Times* **62**: 146.

Pearson K S, Gomez M N, Moyers J R, Carter J G, Tinker J H. (1989) A cost/benefit analysis of randomized invasive monitoring for patients undergoing cardiac surgery. *Anesthesia and Analgesia* **69**: 336–41.

Peckham M. (1991) Research and development for the National Health Service. *Lancet* **338**: 367–71.

Phillips I, Spencer G T. (1965) *Pseudomonas aeruginosa* cross-infection due to contaminated respiratory apparatus. *Lancet* **ii**: 1325–7.

Pickard J. (2008) Obituary: Professor Bryan Jennett. *Independent* (February 16).

Pontoppidan H, Geffin B, Lowenstein E. (1972) Acute respiratory failure in the adult. *New England Journal of Medicine* **287**: 690–8.

Pontoppidan H, Geffin B, Lowenstein E. (1973) *Acute Respiratory Failure in the Adult in 1973*, 1st edn. Boston, MA: Little, Brown.

Postle M. (1971) Faecal peritonitis complicated by severe chest infection – a patient care study. *Nursing Times* **67**: 630–3.

Powell M B. (1966) *The Post-certificate Training and Education of Nurses:* Report by a Sub-Committee of the Standing Nursing Advisory Committee of the Central Health Services Council. London: HMSO.

Powell R. (2007) Withdrawal of treatment: dilemmas in the medical treatment of patients facing inevitable death. *Archives of Disease in Childhood* **92**: 746–9.

Puddicombe M M. (1964) Intensive care unit, Addenbrooke's Hospital, Cambridge. *Nursing Times* **60**: 1030–1.

Quarrell E J. (1970) Artificial ventilation. 3. Nursing care. *Nursing Times* **66**: 1360–2.

Ramsay M A E. (2000) Anesthesia and pain management at Baylor University Medical Center. *Baylor University Medical Center Proceedings* **13**: 151–65.

Ravitsky V. (2005) Timers on ventilators. *British Medical Journal* **330**: 415–17.

Reynolds L A, Tansey E M. (eds) (2000) *Clinical Research in Britain, 1950–80.* Wellcome Witnesses to Twentieth Century Medicine, vol. 7. London: The Wellcome Trust. Freely available online at www.history.qmul.ac.uk/research/modbiomed/wellcome_witnesses/

Reynolds L A, Tansey E M. (eds) (2004) *Innovation in Pain Management.* Wellcome Witnesses to Twentieth Century Medicine, vol. 21. London: The Wellcome Trust Centre for the History of Medicine at UCL. Freely available online at www.history.qmul.ac.uk/research/modbiomed/ wellcome_witnesses/

Reynolds L A, Tansey E M. (eds) (2007) *Medical Ethics Education in Britain, 1963–93.* Wellcome Witnesses to Twentieth Century Medicine, vol. 31. London: The Wellcome Trust Centre for the History of Medicine at UCL. Freely available online at www.history.qmul.ac.uk/research/modbiomed/ wellcome_witnesses/

Reynolds L A, Tansey E M. (eds) (2008a) *Clinical Pharmacology in the UK, c. 1950–2000: Influences and institutions.* Wellcome Witnesses to Twentieth Century Medicine, vol. 33. London: The Wellcome Trust Centre for the History of Medicine at UCL. Freely available online at www.history.qmul.ac.uk/research/modbiomed/ wellcome_witnesses/

Reynolds L A, Tansey E M. (eds) (2008b) *Clinical Pharmacology in the UK, c. 1950–2000: Industry and regulation.* Wellcome Witnesses to Twentieth Century Medicine, vol. 34. London: The Wellcome Trust Centre for the History of Medicine at UCL. Freely available online at www.history.qmul.ac.uk/research/modbiomed/ wellcome_witnesses/

Reynolds L A, Tansey E M. (eds) (2009) *The Development of Sports Medicine in Twentieth-century Britain.* Wellcome Witnesses to Twentieth Century Medicine, vol. 36. London: The Wellcome Trust Centre for the History of Medicine at UCL. Freely available online at www.history.qmul.ac.uk/ research/modbiomed/wellcome_witnesses/

Richardson J C, Ashworth P M. (1966) 'Steak and chips' or tube-feeding without tears. *Nursing Times* **62**: 670–1.

Richmond C. (2005) Obituary: Alan Gilston. *British Medical Journal* **331**: 518.

Richmond C. (2007) Obituary: Bjørn Ibsen. *British Medical Journal* **335**: 674.

Ross D. (1975–77) Looking around in cardiac surgery. Lettsomian lectures I and II. *Transactions of the Medical Society of London* **92–93**: 176–82; 183–91.

Royal College of Nursing. (1969) *The Function and Staffing of Intensive Therapy Units and the Preparation of Nurses to Work in the Units.* London: Royal College of Nursing.

Royle T. (1986) *The Years of Their Lives. The National Service Experience, 1945–63.* London: Michael Joseph.

Russell W R, Schuster E, Crampton Smith A, Spalding J M K. (1956) Radcliffe respiration pumps. *Lancet* **i**: 539–41.

Ryan D W, Copeland P F, Miller J, Freeman R. (1982) Group replanning of an intensive therapy unit. *British Medical Journal* **285**: 1634–7.

Salter M. (1966) Intensive therapy unit: The London Hospital. *Nursing Times* **62**: 1457–60.

Scott C. (1998) Specialist practice: advancing the profession? *Journal of Advanced Nursing* **28**: 554–62.

Severinghaus J W, Astrup P, Murray J F. (1998) Blood gas analysis and critical care medicine. *American Journal of Respiratory and Critical Care Medicine* **157**: S114–22.

Shirley P. (2009) Operational critical care: intensive care and trauma. *Journal of the Royal Army Medical Corps* **155**: 122–74.

Shoemaker W C. (1990) Use and abuse of the balloon tip pulmonary artery (Swan–Ganz) catheter: are patients getting their money's worth? *Critical Care Medicine* **18**: 1294–6.

Siggaard-Andersen O, Engel K, Jorgensen K, Astrup P. (1960) A micro method for determination of pH, carbon dioxide tension, base excess, and standard bicarbonate in capillary blood. *Scandinavian Journal of Clinical and Laboratory Investigation* **12**: 172–6.

Singer M, Grant I. (eds) (1999) *ABC of Critical Care.* Oxford: Wiley-Blackwell.

Singer M, Webb A R. (1997) *Oxford Handbook of Critical Care.* Oxford: Oxford University Press.

Smith A C, Spalding J M K, Russell W R. (1954) Artificial ventilation by intermittent positive pressure in poliomyelitis and other diseases. *Lancet* **i**: 939–45.

Stoddart J C. (1975) *Intensive Therapy.* Oxford: Blackwell Scientific Publications.

Stoddart J C. (1986) A career post – with intensive therapy? *Anaesthesia* **41**: 1181–3.

Stoddart J C. (1994) The development of intensive therapy in the UK. *Current Anaesthesia and Critical Care* **5**: 115–20.

Stoddart J C. (2005) Tribute to Alan Gilston. *Journal of the Intensive Care Society* **6**: 9–11.

Stott S. (2000) Recent advances: recent advances in intensive care. *British Medical Journal* **320**: 358–61.

Swan H J C. (1991) Development of the pulmonary artery catheter. *Disease-a-Month* **37**: 485–508.

Swan H J C. (2005) The pulmonary artery catheter in anesthesia practice. *Anesthesiology* **103**: 890–3.

Swan H J C, Ganz W, Forrester J, Marcus H, Diamond G, Chonette D. (1970) Catheterization of the heart in man with use of a flow-directed balloon-tipped catheter. *New England Journal of Medicine* **283**: 447–51.

Sykes M K. (1960) Intermittent positive pressure respiration in tetanus neonatorum. *Anaesthesia* **15**: 401–10.

Sykes M K. (1962) The East-Radcliffe ventilator adapted for anaesthesia. *British Journal of Anaesthesia* **34**: 203–6.

Sykes M K. (1964) The Anaesthetic Department, Postgraduate Medical School of London and Hammersmith Hospital. *Anesthesia and Analgesia* **43**: 601–9.

Sykes M K. (1988) Ventilator-induced lung damage. *Acta Anaesthesiologica Belgica* **39** (Suppl. 2): 43–4.

Sykes M K. (2008) And so to Boston (1954/5). *International Anesthesiology Clinics* **46**: 199–205.

Sykes M K, Bunker J. (2007) *Anaesthesia and the Practice of Medicine: Historical perspectives*, with John Bunker, contributing editor. London: RSM Press.

Sykes M K, Young J D. (1999) *Respiratory Support in Intensive Care*. London: BMJ Books.

Sykes M K, McNicol M W, Campbell E J M. (1969) *Respiratory Failure*. Oxford: Blackwell Scientific Publications.

Tanner O. (2009) CAT review: intensive versus conventional glucose control in critically ill patients. *Journal of Intensive Care Society* **10**: 216–17.

Tansey E M, Reynolds L A. (eds) (1999) *Early Heart Transplant Surgery in the UK.* Wellcome Witnesses to Twentieth Century Medicine, vol. 3. London: The Wellcome Trust. Freely available online at www.history.qmul.ac.uk/ research/modbiomed/wellcome_witnesses/

Tansey E M, Christie D A. (eds) (2000) *Looking at the unborn: Historical aspects of obstetric ultrasound.* Wellcome Witnesses to Twentieth Century Medicine, vol. 5. London: The Wellcome Trust. Freely available online at www.history. qmul.ac.uk/research/modbiomed/wellcome_witnesses/

Taylor S. (ed.) (1968) *Recent Advances in Surgery.* London: J & A Churchill.

Teasdale G, Jennett W B. (1974) Assessment of coma and impaired consciousness: a practical scale. *Lancet* **304**: 81–4.

Thomas H. (2003) Letter: GMC guidance on withholding life prolonging treatment. *British Medical Journal* **326**: 1215.

Tinker J, Porter S W. (1980) *A Course in Intensive Therapy Nursing.* London: Edward Arnold.

Tobin M J. (ed.) (1994) *Principles and Practice of Mechanical Ventilation.* New York, NY: McGraw-Hill Inc, Health Professions Division.

Trubuhovich R V. (2004) Further commentary on Denmark's 1952/3 poliomyelitis epidemic, especially regarding mortality; with a correction. *Acta Anaesthesiologica Scandinavica* **48**: 1310–15.

Trubuhovich R V. (2006) Notable Australian contributions to the management of ventilatory failure of acute poliomyelitis: with special reference to the Both respirator and Dr John A Forbes. *Critical Care and Resuscitation* **8**: 383–93. Erratum in: *Critical Care and Resuscitation* (2007) **9**: 106.

Trubuhovich R V. (2007a) On the very first, successful, long-term, large-scale use of IPPV. Albert Bower and V Ray Bennett: Los Angeles, 1948–49. *Critical Care and Resuscitation* **9**: 91–100.

Trubuhovich R V. (2007b) History of mouth-to-mouth ventilation. Part 3: the 19th to mid-20th centuries and 'rediscovery'. *Critical Care and Resuscitation* **9**: 221–37.

Tuttle R R, Mills J. (1975) Dobutamine: development of a new catecholamine to selectively increase cardiac contractility. *Circulation Research* **36**: 185–96.

Vincent J-L, Singer M. (2010) Critical care: advances and future perspectives. *Lancet* **376**: 1354–61.

Vincent J-L, Singer M, Marini J J, Moreno R, Levy M, Matthay M A, Pinsky M, Rhodes A, Ferguson N D, Evans T, Annane D, Hall J B. (2010) Thirty years of critical care medicine. *Critical Care* **14**: 311.

Wackers G L. (1994a) Modern anaesthesiological principles for bulbar polio: manual IPPR in the 1952 polio-epidemic in Copenhagen. *Acta Anaesthesiologica Scandinavica* **38**: 420–31.

Wackers G. (1994b) Innovation in artificial respiration: how the 'iron lung' became a museum piece. In Lawrence G. (ed.) *Technologies of Modern Medicine*, proceedings of a seminar held at the Science Museum, London, March 1993. London: Science Museum: 40–57.

Wada J, Iwa T. (eds) *Proceedings of the International Congress on Hyperbaric Medicine.* Tokyo: Igaku Shoin; London: Baillière, Tindall and Cassell.

Waddell G, Scott P D, Lees N W, Ledingham I McA. (1975) Effects of ambulance transport in critically ill patients. *British Medical Journal* **i**: 386–9.

Ward F G. (1970) Rehabilitation in the services I: The Royal Navy. *Rheumatology and Physical Medicine* **10**: 425–8.

Waters R M. (1936) Carbon dioxide absorption from anaesthetic atmospheres. *Proceedings of the Royal Society of Medicine* **30**: 11–22.

Watt I, Ledingham I McA. (1984) Mortality amongst multiple trauma patients admitted to an intensive therapy unit. *Anaesthesia* **39**: 973–81.

Watt I, Fraser R, Kenyon C, Lever A F, Beastall C , Ledingham I McA. (1984) Effect of etomidate on adrenocortical function. *British Journal of Surgery* **71**: 380.

West J B (ed.) (1996) *Respiratory Physiology: People and ideas*, American Physiological Society's People and Ideas series. Oxford: Oxford University Press.

West J B. (2005) The physiological challenges of the 1952 Copenhagen poliomyelitis epidemic and a renaissance in clinical respiratory physiology. *Journal of Applied Physiology* **99**: 424–32.

Wilson M G, Roscoe S N. (1958) Resuscitation of newborn premature infants; a clinical study of the use of positive pressure respiration. *California Medicine* **88**: 312–15.

Working Group on Intensive Care for Respiratory Insufficiency. (1977) *Intensive Care for Respiratory Insufficiency: Report on a working group, Nancy, 21–23 April 1976*, ICP/OCD 003. Copenhagen: Regional Office for Europe, World Health Organization.

Wright D, Mackenzie S J, Buchan I, Cairns C S, Price L E. (1991) Critical incidents in the intensive therapy unit. *Lancet* **338**: 676–8.

Wright R, Sykes M K, Jackson B G, Mann N M, Adams E B. (1961) Intermittent positive pressure respiration in tetanus neonatorum. *Lancet* **ii**: 678–80.

Wyse S D, Pfitzner J, Rees A, Lincoln J C R, Branthwaite M A. (1975) Measurement of cardiac output by thermal dilution in infants and children. *Thorax* **30**: 262–5.

Young J D, Sykes M K. (1990) Assisted ventilation. 1. Artificial ventilation: history, equipment and techniques. *Thorax* **45**: 753–8.

Biographical notes[*]

Ms Sheila Adam
RN BNurs MSc (b. 1957) trained at Manchester University (1975–79) on one of the earliest nursing degree courses. She was appointed as staff nurse to the Royal Free Hospital, London, attended a clinical intensive care course at Guy's Hospital, London, in 1981 and was first appointed as a sister in intensive care at Whipps Cross Hospital, London, in 1983. Appointed senior nurse for intensive care at the Middlesex Hospital, London, in 1985, clinical nurse specialist in 1993 and nurse consultant in expanded critical care in 2000. See also Adam and Osborne (1997).

Dr Aileen Adams
CBE MA FRCS(Eng) FRCA (b. 1923) qualified at Sheffield and spent some of her junior years in anaesthesia at Addenbrooke's Hospital, Cambridge (1946–47; 1949–51); senior registrar, Bristol (1952–55); fellow in anaesthesia, Massachusetts General Hospital, Boston, Massachusetts (1955–57); locum consultant, Oxford (1958/9); senior lecturer, Lagos University Medical School, Nigeria (1963/4), becoming a consultant anaesthetist, Addenbrooke's Hospital, Cambridge (1960–84) and associate lecturer, Cambridge University (1967–84). She has had virtually no experience in intensive care since becoming a consultant. She was dean, Faculty of Anaesthetists, Royal College of Surgeons (1985–88) and president of the History of Anaesthesia Society (1990–92), the History of Medicine Section, Royal Society of Medicine (1994–95) and the British Society for the History of Medicine (2003–05). See her 1996 interview with Dr Max Blythe, held in Oxford Brookes' Medical Sciences Video Archive as MSVA142–3.

Ms Pat Ashworth
SRN SCM MSc FRCN FFNRCSI(Hon) (b. 1930) qualified at Kent County Ophthalmic and Aural Hospital, Maidstone, Guy's Hospital, London, Jessop and Nether Edge Hospitals, Sheffield. Appointed staff nurse, ward sister, night sister at Guy's and elsewhere; sister, cardiothoracic surgery ward, Broadgreen Hospital, Liverpool, 1959, including two ITU beds from (1960) and departmental

[*] Contributors are asked to supply details; other entries are compiled from conventional biographical sources.

sister, in the new ITU (1964–73). She held a DHSS fellowship (1973–76), then joint clinical/academic appointment at the Manchester Royal Infirmary and the University of Manchester (1976–79), one of the first two posts in UK nursing of this kind. She was research programme manager for the Manchester University WHO collaborating centre for nursing (1979–85); and senior lecturer in nursing, University of Ulster (1985–90). Editor of *Intensive Care Nursing/Intensive and Critical Care Nursing* (1985–2000).

Dr Carol Ball

RN MSc PhD (b. 1955) trained as a nurse at the Middlesex Hospital, London (1974–77) with an intensive care course (JBCNS no. 100) at Guy's Hospital. She gained experience in the intensive care unit at the Middlesex Hospital (1980–84), as a staff nurse and sister, with Miss Sue Porter and Dr Jack Tinker. During this time she was awarded a diploma in nursing, University of London (1983). Following the diploma in nurse education, University of London (1985), she was appointed tutor to the intensive care course at St Bartholomew's School of Nursing and Midwifery (1985–93), gaining an MSc in nursing, City University, London (1993) and was appointed course

director to the MSc in nursing studies, City University in the same year. She returned to the field of intensive care as a lecturer, was appointed research fellow (1998), received her PhD in 2000 and was editor-in-chief, *Intensive and Critical Care Nursing*, in the same year. She held a joint appointment as nurse consultant in critical care nursing at the Royal Free Hospital, London (2001) and senior research fellow, later reader in intensive care nursing, City University (2009–10) until her retirement and is immediate past editor of the journal *Intensive Critical Care Nursing*.

Professor Julian Bion

MRCP FRCA FFICM MD (b. 1952) qualified at Charing Cross Hospital, London, trained in general medicine and cardiology, and then in anaesthesia and intensive care medicine. Appointed senior lecturer in intensive care medicine at the University of Birmingham and honorary consultant at the Queen Elizabeth Hospital in 1987, he was promoted to a personal chair of intensive care medicine at the University of Birmingham in 2007 and has been co-director of research and development and deputy director of the Birmingham Clinical Research Academy since 2008. In 2010 he was elected foundation dean of the new Faculty of Intensive Care Medicine for the UK. A member of the Intercollegiate Board, he led the group that wrote the first competency-based training programme for ICM in 2001; was president of the European Society of Intensive Care Medicine (2004–06) and established the European Critical Care Network and led development of the CoBaTrICE programme. He is senior clinical lead for the National Patient Safety Agency project (2009–11) to minimize infections linked to central venous catheters in ICUs throughout England. In 2004 he was presented with the Shubin–Weil award for excellence by the Society of Critical Care Medicine, gave the Gilston lecture and received honorary membership of the Intensive Care Society in 2009.

Professor Ronald Bradley

FRCP (b. 1929), the first person to describe the use of a floating miniature pulmonary artery catheter in man (Bradley (1964)), qualified and trained at St Thomas' Hospital, where he was appointed physician and clinical physiologist in 1965, he was professor of intensive therapy medicine there (1989–95), later emeritus. His extremely narrow catheter was used to determine pulmonary artery pressures and waveforms and later went on to determine thermo dilution cardiac output in man using a thermistor-tipped catheter (Branthwaite and Bradley (1968)), and suggested the use of pulmonary artery-diastolic pressure as an index of mean left atrial pressure (Jenkins *et al.* (1970)).

Dr Margaret Branthwaite

MA FRCP (b. 1935) qualified at Cambridge. Her involvement with intensive care started at the Brompton Hospital in 1963, continued on the surgical unit at St Thomas's Hospital for a year during which she had contact with Dr Bradley who invited her on to the medical unit. Appointed consultant cardiothoracic anaesthetist in intensive care and respiratory medicine at the Brompton Hospital, London (1961–91), she was consultant physician there from 1979 and directed adult intensive care and the respiratory support services, Royal Brompton Hospital, London. She took an MA in medical ethics and law, King's College London in 1989 and retrained as a barrister at Lincoln's Inn in 1993. She has been a non-executive board member of UK Transplant's special health board and her 1997 interview with Lady Wendy Ball is held in Oxford Brookes' Medical Sciences Video Archive as MSVA170. See also Branthwaite (2000).

Dr Doreen Browne

FFA RCS MSc (anthropology) FRCA (b. 1934) qualified at the Royal Free Hospital Medical School and obtained her fellowship of the Faculty of Anaesthetists of the Royal College of Surgeons in 1966. Appointed research fellow at the respiratory care unit, Massachusetts General Hospital, Boston, in 1970/1, with a special interest in weaning patients from mechanical ventilation, she was consultant anaesthetist at the Royal Free in 1971, with one ITU session, subsequently increased to three. Senior lecturer to Benin, Nigeria, for six months (1973) to help set up an ITU there. Returning to London, she became a member of the Intensive Care Society, regional education adviser in anaesthesia and intensive care in the NHS NE Thames region; examiner for the fellowship in anaesthesia and was elected a member of the council of the Royal Colleges of Anaesthesia (1990–98).

Dr Anthony (Tony) Gilbertson

FRCA (b. 1932) qualified from Liverpool in 1956 and trained there as an anaesthetist under Professor Cecil Gray and Dr Jackson Rees. After service in the medical branch of the Royal Air Force (1959–64), he was appointed consultant in Sefton General Hospital, Liverpool in 1966 and established an ITU there, specializing in the management of combined respiratory and renal failure and director of that unit and the unit at the Royal Liverpool Hospital until 1989. He has held several offices, including associate dean and vice-president of the Royal Society of Medicine, president of Liverpool Society of Anaesthetists, the Liverpool division of the British Medical Association and was a visiting professor at McGill University (1980–82). He was elected a distinguished member of the Intensive Care Society in 1998.

Professor Sir Ian Gilmore

Kt MD PRCP (b. 1947) trained at Cambridge and St Thomas' and after various house jobs, including SHO on the intensive therapy unit, St Thomas' Hospital (1973) and registrar in general medicine and gastroenterology there (1974/5), was an MRC research fellow in the gastrointestinal lab at Charing Cross Hospital. Appointed consultant physician and gastroenterologist at Royal Liverpool and Broadgreen Hospitals Liverpool (1980–), where he was medical director (1995–98); directed R&D at the Royal Liverpool University Hospital (1993–95) and honorary lecturer in the department of medicine at the University of Liverpool (1980–98), being chairman of the faculty of medicine (1991/2) and professor (1999–); and chairman of the Standing Liaison Committee, Mersey Regional Health Authority and the University of Liverpool (1991–94). He chaired a Royal College of Physicians working party on alcohol misuse in 2001. He was president of the Royal College of Physicians (2006–10).

Dr Alan Gilston

FRCS(Eng) FFARCS (1928–2005) was senior consultant anaesthetist at the National Heart Hospital (1967–90). A former president and founder of the World Federation of Societies of Intensive and Critical Care Medicine, secretary-general and initiator of the First World Congress on Intensive Care in 1974 and chairman and founder of the Intensive Care Society; he gave the first Gilston lecture and was Silver Medallist of the Society. See Richmond (2005); Stoddart (2005).

Mr Graham Haynes

SRN RSCN DipTH PGCE MSc (b. 1950) trained at Leicester Royal Infirmary, with intensive care training at Westminster Hospital, London and training in tropical health at London School of Hygiene and Tropical Medicine (1972/3) and in child nursing at Great Ormond Street Hospital (1982/3). Appointed night and day charge nurse, Westminster Hospital (1973–

75), charge nurse, ITU, Middlesex Hospital, London (1975–77), night nursing officer, Westminster Hospital (1977/8), nursing officer for ITU services (CCU, RICU and CTU), Westminster Hospital (1978–81). He was tutor to the neonatal intensive care services course (1981–85); the intensive care course, St Thomas' Hospital (1985/6), senor tutor for specialist courses, the Nightingale School, London (1986–89), head of post-registration programmes, Nightingale School (1989–91), head of continuing professional studies for nurses, Guy's and Nightingale Schools of Nursing (1991–93), senior lecturer in child health nursing, King's College London (1993–2005). He was an advisor to UNICEF (2006), and to the Tropical Health Education Trust (2006–09).

Professor Peter Hutton

PhD FRCA FRCP FIMechE (b. 1947) qualified in medicine in 1978, following an initial career in mechanical engineering and bioengineering research. He was professor of anaesthesia at the University of Birmingham and honorary consultant at the University Hospital, Birmingham (1986–2010), president of the Royal College of Anaesthetists (2000–03) and chairman of the Academy of Medical Royal

Colleges (2002–04). He is also a chartered engineer. He has been an external consultant in clinical governance for NHS organizations; an assessor for the National Clinical Assessment Service; a member of the General Medical Council, and is currently the independent consultant member of the Prescription Medicines Code of Practice Appeal Board. Until 2010, he chaired a non-departmental public body advising on the ethical aspects of forensic DNA and was a lay member of the Bar Standards Board (2007–10). He is the anaesthesia adviser on the National Clinical Assessment Team and founder director of the FH Partnership Ltd, established to promote quality and improve cost effectiveness in healthcare.

Professor Bjørn Ibsen
(1915–2007), anaesthetist and intensivist, was senior resident (reservelaege, anaesthesiology), department of surgery I, Rigshospitalet, Kommunehospitalet, Copenhagen (1953/4) and professor of anaesthesiology and chief of department, University of Copenhagen (1954–71). He opened and supervised the first ITU in the Kommunehospitalet in 1953 until his interests moved towards pain management in 1975. See Richmond (2007).

Professor Bryan Jennett
CBE MD FRCS (1926–2008) qualified at Liverpool University Medical School, trained at Oxford with Sir Hugh Cairns and at the RAMC Military Hospital, Wheatley. Appointed lecturer in neurosurgery at the University of Manchester (1957–63); Rockefeller fellow at the University of California at Los Angeles (UCLA); appointed consultant neurosurgeon in Glasgow in 1963, and became foundation professor of neurosurgery, University of Glasgow in 1968. Member of the Medical Research Council (1974–77); dean of the Faculty of Medicine (1981–85); president of the section of neurology, Royal Society of Medicine (1986/7); and president of the International Society of Technology Assessment in Health Care (1987–89). See Pickard (2008).

Professor Desmond Laurence
FRCP (b. 1922) qualified in medicine from St Thomas' Hospital Medical School, London, in 1944 and was appointed lecturer in therapeutics there in 1950; senior lecturer in pharmacology and therapeutics at University College Hospital Medical School jointly with University College London (1954–61) and professor there (1961–89); served on the Committee on Safety of Drugs,

Committee on Safety of Medicines and the Medicines Commission (1963–88). In 1967 he was a member of the Royal College of Physicians' committee on the supervision of the ethics of clinical investigations and institutions, and subsequently served on the college's Committee on Ethical Issues in Medicine. For 26 years he served on research ethics committees as chairman or member.

Professor Iain Ledingham

MSc (Hons) MD (Hons) FRCS FRCP FACCM FInstBiol DMI FRSE (b. 1935), qualified at Glasgow University Medical School, trained at the Western Infirmary, Glasgow with Professors Sir Charles Illingworth and Sir Andrew Kay, appointed to the Hall fellowship in surgery (1960), proceeding to reader in surgery and consultant in intensive care (1973) and professor of intensive care medicine (1980–88). He became professor of emergency and critical care medicine, Faculty of Medicine and Health Sciences United Arab Emirates University (1988) and thereafter dean (1989–95). On return to the UK, he was appointed director of the health care learning network and chair of medical education, University of Dundee (1995–2000). He was the first president of the UK Intensive Care Society (1972–74) and its first honorary life member; president of the European Society of Intensive Care Medicine (1990–92); president of the European Shock Society (1983–85) and WHO/EC Consultant in acute care medicine (1973–2005). He was made the first UK fellow of the American College of Critical Care Medicine in 1991.

Ms Alice Nicholls

(b. 1975) is a PhD student at the Centre for the History of Science, Technology and Medicine, University of Manchester. Her forthcoming thesis is titled 'Life in the balance: critical illness and British intensive care, 1948–99'.

Professor Mervyn Singer

MD FRCP FRCP (Edin) (b. 1958) qualified at St Bartholomew's Hospital Medical College and trained in general medicine and intensive care at various hospitals in and around London. He has been professor of intensive care medicine at UCL since 2001 and has published widely and written or edited several textbooks. He was the first UK intensivist to be awarded senior investigator status by the National Institute for Health Research. See Singer and Webb (1997); Singer and Grant (eds) (1999).

Dr Brian Slawson

FFA RCS Eng (b. 1933) qualified in Edinburgh and trained in anaesthetics at the Royal Infirmary, Edinburgh. Appointed MRC scientific assistant, department of therapeutics (1962/3), university lecturer in anaesthesia, University of Edinburgh (1963–66), he was consultant anaesthetist, Western General Hospital, Edinburgh, and honorary senior lecturer in anaesthesia (1966–94) and at the Eastern General Hospital, Edinburgh (1994–98).

Dr Geoffrey Tallent Spencer

OBE FFARCS (b. 1929) qualified at St Thomas' Hospital, London, and trained there and at Southampton. In 1962 he was a senior registrar and was appointed to plan a new multidisciplinary purpose-built ten-bed ITU and two years later was appointed as consultant anaesthetist to run the new St. Thomas' Hospital's intensive care unit, which he did until his retirement in 1994. He was appointed consultant-in-charge of the long-term respiratory unit, St. Thomas' Hospital, in 1968. He has also been a WHO consultant (1973); visiting professor at the Children's Memorial Hospital, Chicago, (1976); honorary consultant to the Brompton Hospital (1982–92). He was deputy chairman of the BMA's working party on intensive care (BMA Planning Unit (1967)). He was appointed OBE in 1982 by the Queen for 'Services to Disabled people'.

Dr Joseph Stoddart

MD FRCA FRCP (b. 1932) qualified at Durham and served in the RAF medical branch (1960–65), RAF Institute of Aviation Medicine, high altitude division (1963–65). He was first assistant to Professor E A Pask, department of anaesthetics, University of Newcastle upon Tyne. He was appointed consultant in anaesthetics and director of intensive therapy, Royal Victoria Infirmary, Newcastle (1967–95) and was founder member and one-time chairman of the Intensive Care Society; a member of council and examiner, Royal College of Anaesthetics; a member of the National Confidential Enquiry into Patient Outcome and Death; chairman of the Intercollegiate Committee for Intensive Care, and honorary life member of the Intensive Care Society.

Professor Leo Strunin

MD FRCA FRCPC (b. 1937) qualified at Durham University and trained in Newcastle. He entered the academic track in 1965 at the London Hospital Medical College and in 1976 took up the chair of anaesthetics at King's College Hospital Medical School, moving to Canada in 1980 to head the academic department of anaesthesia, University of Calgary, Alberta, Canada. He returned to England in 1990 and took up the BOC chair of anaesthesia at Barts and The Royal London, Queen Mary's School of Medicine and Dentistry, Queen Mary, University of London, until his retirement in 2003, later emeritus. He was a member of council of the Royal College of Anaesthetists (RCA) in 1992 and served as president (1997–2000) and was president of the Association of Anaesthetists of Great Britain and Ireland (AAGBI) (2000–02). He was postgraduate issue editor of the *British Journal of Anaesthesia* (1991–96).

Professor Sir Keith Sykes

FFARCS HonFANZCA HonFCA (SA) 1989 (b. 1925) qualified at Magdalene College, Cambridge, and after anaesthetic training in the Royal Army Medical Corps, University College Hospital and the Massachusetts General Hospital, Boston, Massachusetts, he was appointed lecturer in anaesthesia and consultant anaesthetist, Postgraduate Medical School, Hammersmith Hospital, London (1958–67), becoming a reader in 1967 and professor of clinical anaesthesia in 1970. From 1980–91

he was Nuffield professor of anaesthetics at the University of Oxford. He was knighted in 1991 and became an Honorary Fellow of Pembroke College, Oxford in 1996. In 1959 he spent six months in the King Edward VIII Hospital, Durban, South Africa, initiating a controlled trial of mechanical ventilation in the treatment of neonatal tetanus. On his return to Hammersmith Hospital he set up an in-hospital cardiac arrest service, a blood gas service, and anaesthetized patients for open heart surgery. In 1960 he initiated the use of postoperative mechanical ventilation and developed an intensive care unit that he ran until 1969. He has written books on the treatment of respiratory failure, clinical measurement and the history of anaesthesia. See his 1997 interview with Lady Wendy Ball, held in Oxford Brookes' Medical Sciences Video Archive as MSVA159.

Professor Tilli Tansey

PhD PhD HonMRCP HonFRCP FMedSci (b. 1953) is convenor of the History of Twentieth Century Medicine Group and professor of the history of modern medical sciences at Queen Mary, University of London.

Dr Jack Tinker

FRCP FRCS Glasgow (1936–2010) qualified at Manchester and trained as a cardiothoracic surgeon at

Manchester Royal Infirmary, later switching to cardiology and general medicine. He caught hepatitis B from a dialysis patient in 1966, was in a coma for 48 hours and survived, receiving treatment from Sheila Sherlock. He switched to research and worked for Sir James Black at ICI Pharmaceuticals on the development of β-blockers (1967–69), moving to London in 1969 when appointed as a lecturer at the Royal Postgraduate Medical School, Hammersmith Hospital. In 1986 he became dean of postgraduate medicine in the North East Thames Regional Health Authority, where he instituted training programmes for house officers and junior medical staff and in retirement worked at the Royal Society of Medicine, including as dean (1998–2002). He was founding editor of the *European Journal of Intensive Care Medicine* and editor of the *British Journal of Hospital Medicine* (1984–2010). See Fricker (2010).

Dr David Wright

FRCA (b. 1944) qualified in 1968 at St Bartholomew's Hospital, London, trained in anaesthesia at Plymouth General Hospital, St Bartholomew's Hospital, London, and Edinburgh's Royal Infirmary. He was consultant anaesthetist with an interest in intensive care at the Western General Hospital, Edinburgh (1979–2005).

Dr Harold Youngman

MD FFARCS DA (1900–1984) qualified at the University of Cambridge and St Thomas' Hospital, gaining an MD with a thesis on insulin and metabolism, followed by a year at Bellevue Hospital, New York, before entering general practice in Cambridge and honorary anaesthetist and clinical assistant in ophthalmology and paediatrics at Addenbrooke's Hospital. His interests included tetanus and the use of curare, and he established an artificial respiration unit. He became a consultant at the start of the NHS while retaining his general practice. He treated patients with chronic intractable pain and those in terminal care, started a pre-anaesthetic clinic and started postgraduate education in anaesthesia in 1950s Cambridge. See AA *et al.* (1985).

Index: Subject

Index: Names

Biographical notes appear in bold

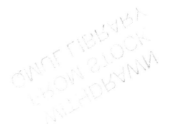

Key to cover photographs

Front cover, left to right

Professor Ronald Bradley

Dr Tony Gilbertson

Dr David Wright

Dr Margaret Branthwaite

Professor Sir Keith Sykes

Back cover, left to right

Professor Iain Ledingham

Ms Pat Ashworth

Dr Geoffrey Spencer

Dr Aileen Adams

Professor Peter Hutton (chair)

Lightning Source UK Ltd.
Milton Keynes UK
UKOW030206071011

179861UK00001B/12/P